WELL-LEADER MINDSET INVESTMENT GUIDE

WELL-LEADER MINDSET INVESTMENT GUIDE

Essential Guide to
OPTIMIZE YOUR HEALTH &
WELLNESS ROI

LORI LINDBERGH, PHD

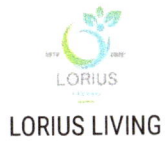

LORIUS LIVING

CONTENTS

Printed in the United States of America

Paperback ISBN: 978-1-958714-70-6

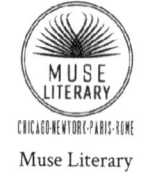

Muse Literary
3319 N. Cicero Avenue
Chicago IL 60641-9998

DISCLAIMER & USE

Disclaimer

The information, standards, and research presented in this guide are current as of the publication date. The author is providing education and information to assist you with improving your personal health and wellness. To receive full benefit, use this guide as a companion resource for this author's book: WELL-LEADER MINDSET: **OPTIMIZE YOUR HEALTH & WELLNESS ROI.**

It is up to you to use your own judgment before applying any information in your own life. The author is not guaranteeing specific results and is not responsible for you misapplying the information in your own life. The author is not a medical doctor, therapist, or counselor. She is not diagnosing and not giving medical, nutritional, and mental health advice or recommendations. Should you need further support, the author will provide resources to assist you with an appropriate referral should your situation fall outside her scope of practice.

It is your responsibility to always seek medical advice/clearance and discuss all health, nutrition, and lifestyle changes with your healthcare providers and/or licensed counselor before you implement any changes.

Copyright & Use

The author is providing the information and resources in this guide for your personal, non-commercial use. You may not in any way use, copy, adapt, or represent that her content is yours or created by you.

After subscribing to the book resource website at www.well-leadermindset.com, you may download and print the forms and resources for your personal use but cannot use or reproduce any of the content for your own business purposes or wellness coaching practice use, nor are you authorized to distribute electronic files downloaded from the book resource website to others without written permission of the author.

You must submit an email request to the author for permission to use the content in this guide, the book, and the book resource website for use other than your personal improvement and development. Please send your email requests to **lori@loriuslifestyle.com.**

NOTE: WELL-LEADER MINDSET™ trademark registration by LORIUS Lifestyle is in progress at the time of this publication.

WELCOME

The future you as a Well-Leader is right in front of you. Step forward into your authentic wellness today!

WELCOME to the WELL-LEADER MINDSET™ – *Lifestyle Wellness Strategic Plan* development process, your **strategic planning** process to begin your journey toward authentic lifestyle wellness.

I am happy you decided to invest in your wellness and focus on yourself as you begin your mindset transformation toward achieving the health and wellness you desire! I am here to support you in any way I can.

As a leader, you are familiar with how strategic planning supports success and guides the direction of your organization. The same is true for your wellness. As you complete your reading and strategic wellness activities, you assemble the components of your *Lifestyle Wellness Strategic Plan* to guide your WELL-LEADER MINDSET™ **Strategic Progression**.

On a personal note, I am honored to support your journey toward the authentic health and wellness you envision. As you may know, I was an unwell leader for over thirty years, trying just about everything to achieve the health and wellness I desired. Nothing seemed to work, and the extreme diets and programs I tried were not sustainable. I finally cracked the code I'm sharing with you in my book and this investment guide.

I feel confident you will find what works for you to achieve and maintain the wellness you desire now and for the rest of your life. But first, you get to step back, forget what you think you know about health and wellness, and open your mind to endless possibilities. Then, you commit to *Doing the Book* using this investment guide and complete all activities fully to set yourself up to optimize your health and wellness ROI now and long into the future.

For further support, please join me in my LinkedIn group: Well-Leader Mindset™ - The 3% Club, to collaborate with other like-minded Well-Leaders, submit questions, and access additional tips and resources to enhance your wellness strategic planning experience.

Most of all, have fun, relax, and immerse yourself in envisioning your strategic wellness journey of a lifetime!

Dr. Lori
Your Wellness Investment Strategist

HOW TO USE THE WLM INVESTMENT GUIDE

Live & Do the book for the next twelve weeks

"Knowing is not enough; we must apply. Willingness is not enough; we must do."

-BRUCE LEE

This investment guide is essential for you to experience authentic wellness and optimize your health and wellness ROI. It contains information, worksheets, and resources to support creating your *Lifestyle Wellness Strategic Plan*, becoming a Well-Leader, and investing in your wellness for life.

I've organized this guide to align with a twelve-week completion timeline. Following this timeline provides enough time to read the book chapters, complete and practice the associated strategic wellness activities, and foster deeper thinking and the mindset shift necessary for you to become a **savvy wellness investor**.

I recommend you commit to developing your *Lifestyle Wellness Strategic Plan* over twelve weeks because this seems to be the sweet spot for most leaders. Any shorter, you don't have time to complete and reflect on the activities fully; any longer, work and life will get in your way.

Finding your authentic wellness takes time, patience, and diligence. Lifestyle wellness is not a race or a quick-fix solution. Completing the activities in this guide creates a solid foundation to build upon to achieve optimal wellness for the rest of your life.

You can complete most of the strategic wellness activities using the forms in this guide; however, **I highly suggest downloading the fillable PDF forms for all worksheets.** These are available on the book resource website at www.well-leadermindset.com. Enter your email to access the resource website, and bookmark the site for future access.

You will also receive weekly emails containing wellness investment guidance, links to WLM group strategy sessions, and advice to support your twelve-week journey and beyond. Be sure to add my email to your safe list.

The planning process presented in the book is an immersive, intense experience, not a quick weekend read. Your wellness is one of your most important projects, so why not take the next twelve weeks to plan and design your authentic wellness—the wellness you decide feels real, effortless, and genuine to you?

To fully engage in the process and reap the benefits, I suggest you commit 3-5 hours per week to complete the chapter readings and strategic wellness activities, plus time to apply and practice new actions and behaviors at home and work. Some of the activities and reflections may seem a bit quirky and unusual. There is a method to my madness, and my process is backed by science.

You are learning a new way of believing and thinking about your health and wellness. Questions will arise. At the end of each chapter, I've included a space to take notes and write down questions that need answering.

Feel free to post your questions in my LinkedIn group, share in a **WLM group strategy session**, or submit your questions confidentially using the form on the book resource website. You are not alone; my support is always a post, email, or strategy session away.

DAVID'S T-7 APHORISM

You get to: Take the Time to Take the Time

My husband's T-7 Aphorism always echoes in my brain when I embark on a new project or journey: You Must *Take the Time to Take the Time*! I still must remind myself that my wellness is not a race. I'm invested for life. The most important thing is taking the time to find your authentic path forward.

This investment guide is essential to taking the time to complete the *Lifestyle Wellness Strategic Plan* development process presented in the book. It supports your transformation to thinking and believing as a Well-Leader. You learn how to think more strategically and long-term about how to invest, achieve, maintain, and defend the lifelong wellness you desire and believe is possible now.

It takes time for you to practice and shift your mindset, fight through the uncomfortableness, and silence your limitations to open your mind to create a custom strategic wellness plan that feels authentic for your lifestyle. **Your plan must feel right for you.**

The planning process may seem intense. However, it needs to be. This process is about you making critical life-and-death decisions using your lifestyle choices. You are focusing on a well-life for the rest of your life.

One of your most significant projects is your health and wellness. So, step back and *take the time to take the time* to plan it out! Effective planning requires focused thought and time. Documenting your plan brings your thinking to the forefront and increases your success. Failing to plan is planning to fail!

Lifestyle transformation takes time and inspired practice. Your authentic wellness will soon become your way of life. Commit to taking the time to invest in your health and wellness and create your plan over the next twelve weeks!

Becoming a lifelong health-seeker requires perseverance, resilience, and commitment. These are characteristics you already possess as an effective leader. Leverage these characteristics and your innate strengths and values to do what it takes to become the best version of yourself for life. Add years to your life and life to your years!

Let's Get Started!

WEEK 1

YOUR HEALTH & WELLNESS DESTINY IS YOURS TO DEFEND

Fight back against the root cause of chronic diseases – Your Lifestyle!

Only 3% of adults in the US practice healthy levels of four critical health behaviors (non-smoking, healthy weight management, regular movement, and balanced nutrition)

-AMERICAN COLLEGE OF LIFESTYLE MEDICINE

Is your brain up for the task? A recent research study found that even though leaders may be somewhat healthier than the average American, their cognitively demanding jobs increase the need for effective lifestyle medicine strategies (S. McDowell-Larsen, 2021). So who just wants to be **somewhat healthier than average**?

Also cited in the article, as of 2017, 60% of adults in the US were suffering from at least one chronic condition of lifestyle (diabetes, obesity, heart disease, cancer, kidney disease, etc.) and 42% with multiple conditions. And average waist circumference in the study population was 4% higher than average. **It still sounds a bit *squishy* to me.**

Where are you with your health and wellness? Are you not budging much, still a bit *squishy*, making good progress, or well on your way toward extraordinary health and wellness?

Mindset change is the first step to genuinely achieving the health and wellness you desire. Mindset change begins by viewing your health and wellness from a strategic perspective. Next, you commit to your WELL-LEADER MINDSET™ **Strategic Progression**.

In **Week 1**, you get to **give yourself permission** to make your health and wellness a priority and **find your *Why*** that keeps you focused on your wellness for life.

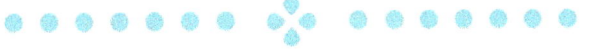

INTRODUCTION

IT STARTS WITH A WAKE-UP CALL

There is no better time than now to start living a healthy life.

Get ready for the first day of your new life. **It's never too late to start living a healthier you**; however, sooner rather than later is much better. The sooner you take charge, the greater your potential to manage, reverse, and prevent the development of chronic diseases of lifestyle, even those that may run in your family.

When I experienced my wake-up call, my brain automatically went into **victim mode**. I blamed everything else and everyone under the sun for my *unwellness*. After the initial shock and anger, I focused on regret about squandered opportunities and *should haves*. This may be what you are experiencing now.

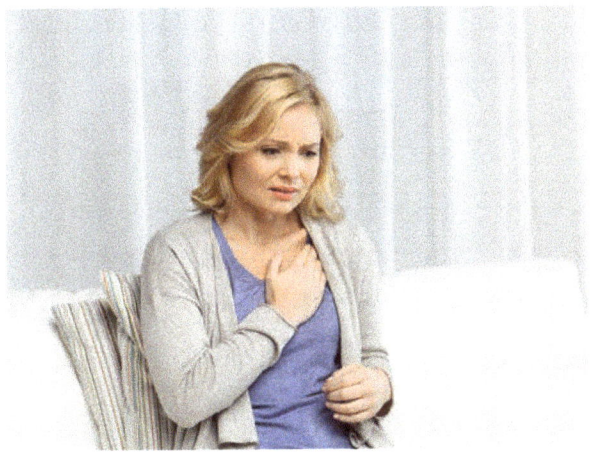

Are you experiencing your wake-up call? What makes it different this time?

It's called **negativity bias.** Our brains naturally go to the negative when we experience a stressful situation. Your brain wants you hyperfocused on the negative, which is not always helpful, but we are wired for survival. If you remember the negative and all the danger, you stay alive longer, right?

When you experience your wake-up call, you do need *saving* **to stay alive longer; however, your negativity bias tends to have the opposite effect.** Instead of taking action to protect yourself, you may avoid the negativity or rely on unhealthy coping mechanisms to distract and medicate, further sabotaging your health and well-being.

Today is the day you STOP perpetuating your negativity bias by understanding where it is coming from so you can reconstruct your thoughts and rewire your brain.

Strategic Wellness Activities

It's time to rip the bandage off and get moving. Like me, you may have been here before, experiencing an intense emotional breakdown or a period of extreme frustration or disgust. You may have just learned about a health condition or suffered a health scare. Often it takes something like this for some people to pull their heads out of the sand.

1. **Access the book resource website.**

You can access the book resource website at www.well-leadermindset.com or use the QR Code.

Enter your email address to receive the link and weekly email support, tips, wellness advising, and access to fillable PDF versions of all forms from the guide should you prefer to complete your plan development work electronically. **Be sure to add my email to your safe list.**

2. **Complete the reflective writing activity.**

You may have experienced a wake-up call recently or had previous experiences that felt like wake-up calls. But, if you are here today, for some reason, these experiences didn't motivate you to change or didn't stick. This is normal. However, something is different this time.

    a. Describe your current wake-up call.

_____

_____

_____

    b. What makes this time different than before? What makes this your real wake-up call and your *not-me* moment?

_____

_____

_____

You can experience cognitive dissonance with your health and wellness and in other areas of your life. By working through this program and stepping into your authentic wellness, you can, and you will end your wellness cognitive dissonance.

How do you know when it has ended? **It ends when you achieve health and wellness authenticity.** You no longer hear yourself saying (aloud or in thought), "I should…, I shouldn't…, I know this isn't healthy but…, I'm being bad, I'm lazy, etc." These are just thoughts. You have believed them and repeated them so often that they sound factual to you.

Achieving your authentic wellness ends the dissonance by aligning your behaviors with your desired health and wellness to fit your desired lifestyle. **As a result, you truly believe in and live your effortless new way of life.**

NOTES & QUESTIONS TO BE ANSWERED

| 1 |

Give Yourself the Gift of Wellness

No amount of action can override limiting beliefs.

Decision fatigue, doubt, and all kinds of things creep in when you're not paying attention, which keep you stuck in the chasm of inaction. This is especially true for your health and wellness.

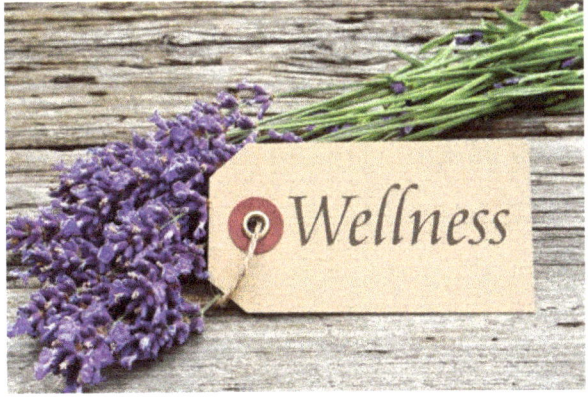

Your wellness is a gift from you to you!

You've made an important decision to take the time to focus on yourself for the next twelve weeks. As you begin your wellness journey of a lifetime, you get to transform your mindset into one that believes in and supports achieving the health and wellness you desire!

You must pull the weeds (struggles & limiting beliefs) out at the root, or they keep growing back. Think of it as pruning and clipping the hedges and weeds in your brain. You do this by shifting your mindset.

You don't need a new day to start over; you only need a new mindset.

Strategic Wellness Activities

It's time to commit. How and when do you get to show up for yourself? Just as you do in your work, you must commit the time to achieve the wellness you desire. Think about the best time(s) for you to complete your Lifestyle Wellness Strategic Plan development activities.

Only you can complete the activities—no delegating. Document your commitment to yourself for the next twelve weeks. How and when do you get to show up for yourself to begin shifting your mindset?

1. Review your primary calendar.

Then, schedule 3-5 hours weekly to read the book chapters, reflect, and complete the *Lifestyle Wellness Strategic Plan* development activities. Try scheduling shorter time chunks throughout the week. Finding what you can consistently commit to each week is the most important thing.

> **The days/times I commit to working on my *Lifestyle Wellness Strategic Plan* development activities are:**
>
> _____
>
> _____

2. Plan for work and life getting in the way.

Identify 1-2 techniques you will use to help you stay committed to the time you have blocked off in your schedule. If you have an assistant, ask your assistant to schedule your you-time and support your strategic wellness journey.

> **The techniques I will use to keep myself motivated and committed to my wellness meetings with myself are:**
>
> _____
>
> _____
>
> _____
>
> _____

3. Complete the Courage & Confidence Check.

It takes **courage** and **confidence** to achieve and maintain the wellness you desire. As a busy leader, being pulled in multiple directions is a typical day for you. It's easy to get distracted and put your wellness on hold when feeling overwhelmed, stressed, or constrained by tight work deadlines.

> Using a scale of 1-10 (with 10 being Extremely High and 1 being Extremely Low), what are your **courage** and **confidence** levels with **your ability to commit the time and show up for yourself** to achieve the health and wellness you desire?
>
> My **courage** level is:
>
> 1   2   3   4   5   6   7   8   9   10
>
> My **confidence** level is:
>
> 1   2   3   4   5   6   7   8   9   10

What influenced my rating choices?

_____

_____

If my ratings are less than 7, I will take the following actions to increase my **courage** and **confidence**:

_____

_____

4. Create your reflective journal entries to begin building your self-awareness.

By turning your attention inward through journaling, you can become more aware of your traits, behaviors, feelings, beliefs, values, and motivations. Becoming more self-aware can increase your confidence and can help you make better decisions aligned with your long-term health and wellness goals.

a. **What are my thoughts and beliefs about getting started with the _Lifestyle Wellness Strategic Plan_ development process?**

_____

_____

_____

b. **What support do I believe I need to be successful? What options are available for the support I desire?**

_____

_____

_____

c. **What thoughts, feelings, & concerns am I having that are creating resistance and need to be cleaned up to move forward?**

_____

_____

_____

5. Collaborate with Well-Leader peers and get additional support.

Join me and other Well-Leaders in my LinkedIn group: Well-Leader Mindset™ - The 3% Club.

NOTES & QUESTIONS TO BE ANSWERED

| 2 |

Seize the Movement

You don't get what you want in life; you get who you are!

You've committed to an unknown future and to step out of your comfort zone, which can often feel frightening and overwhelming! But instead of fear and uncertainty, **focus on knowing it is possible for you to influence the expression of your genes and boost your immunity through self-care!**

Change starts in your brain, and your subconscious brain controls 95 percent of your thinking - your subconscious brain wants to avoid pain, seek pleasure, and conserve energy. So, it's no wonder willpower rarely works in the long term.

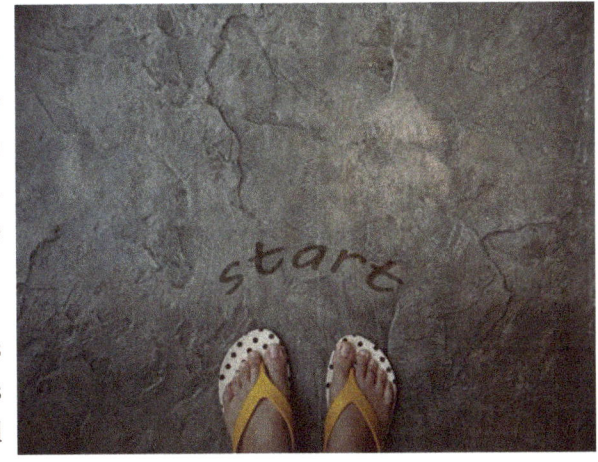

You get to begin taking care of yourself now!

Your brain is wired to avoid making wellness changes that cause discomfort and instead seeks pleasurable ways to medicate yourself with food and alcohol and send you to the couch to binge-watch after a stressful day.

A possibilities mindset knows how to use the other 5 percent of your brain, the prefrontal cortex, to consciously overpower the subconscious. But you need to know what you are dealing with first.

Strategic Wellness Activities

You get to begin taking care of yourself and potentially treating, reversing, and stopping chronic diseases of lifestyle from becoming your destiny! Are you ready to accept the challenge and seize the movement?

1. Complete the reflective writing activity.

Think for a minute about why you are finally ready to take care of yourself and give yourself the gift of health and wellness now.

> **a. Why now? I am ready to change my thinking and give myself the gift of wellness now because:**
>
> _____
>
> _____
>
> _____
>
> **b. How can I think differently about any resistance and self-imposed limitations so I can finally seize my health and wellness movement?**
>
> _____
>
> _____
>
> _____

2. Complete the free WELL-LEADER MINDSET™ **Profile Snapshot evaluation.**

Your current mindset influences your thinking about making a strategic investment to achieve the health and wellness you desire.

Find out how your mindset supports and, at the same time, may limit your progress toward achieving your health and wellness goals.

> NOTE: Access the WLM Profile Snapshot evaluation in the Week 1 section on the book resource website or use this QR code.

Complete your evaluation

3. Complete the Courage & Confidence Check.

It's essential to check in with yourself often to examine your thinking and feelings along the way. It takes **courage** and **confidence** to take the first steps to seize your wellness movement. Also, chapter readings and activities may raise new thoughts, feelings, and concerns to work through.

a. Using a scale of 1-10 (with 10 being Extremely High and 1 being Extremely Low), what are your **courage** and **confidence** levels with your **ability to seize the movement and commit to giving yourself the gift of health and wellness**?

My current **courage** level is:

1   2   3   4   5   6   7   8   9   10

My current **confidence** level is:

1   2   3   4   5   6   7   8   9   10

What influenced my rating choices?

_____

_____

If my ratings are less than 7, I will take the following actions to increase my **courage** and **confidence**:

_____

_____

b. Your **courage** and **confidence** are affected by your readiness to commit to making changes. You may feel courageous and confident, but are you truly ready?

Using a scale of 1-10 (with 10 being Extremely Ready and 1 being Not Ready At All), what is your **readiness to give yourself the gift of wellness**?

My current **readiness** level is:

1   2   3   4   5   6   7   8   9   10

What influenced my rating choice?

_____

_____

If my rating is less than 7, I will take the following actions to increase my **readiness**:

_____

_____

NOTES & QUESTIONS TO BE ANSWERED

| 3 |

Why Now? Uncover Your True Wellness Why

The greatest gift you can give your family and the world is a healthy you.

To jumpstart your strategic wellness journey, you must **take time to find the true *Wellness Why* driving your desire for health and wellness now and into the future**. Your true *Wellness Why* creates the energy you need to finally make the shift in the direction you want to go.

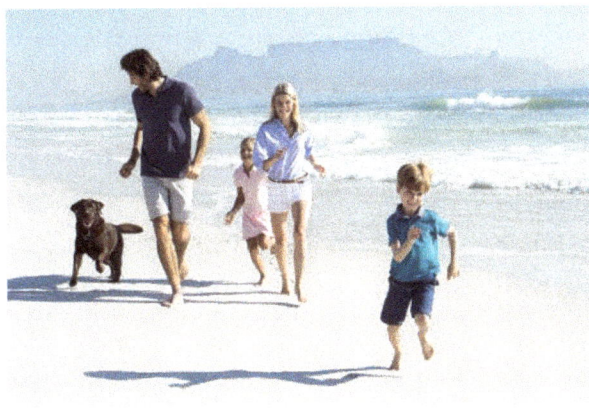

When you find your true Wellness Why, you will know it!

***Wellness Whys* are formatted as "*I desire*" statements, framed in a POSITIVE light.**

Your statements focus on **what you gain** when you change your thinking and achieve the health and wellness you desire.

Focus on what you desire, not what you want. Focusing on *want* creates more negative emotions and puts your brain into a constant state of not having.

Desire is more about setting an intention or belief, which creates more "gentleness" around our perspective and is an easier place to be. If your *Wellness Why* does not make you cry or experience an emotional response, keep looking!

Strategic Wellness Activities

You will use the **5-Whys for problem-solving technique** to uncover your true *Wellness Why*. If you are not familiar with the 5-Whys technique, there are several YouTube® videos available to view the technique in action for problem-solving.

NOTE: A link to a video is in the Week 1 section on the book resource website.

1. Create a safe space to uncover your true *Wellness Why*.

Set aside **thirty minutes** to complete this activity. Find a quiet place free from distractions. Take five deep cleansing breaths in through your nose and out through your mouth. Then rub your hands together for a few seconds to connect your creative and analytical brain areas.

Close your eyes and clear your mind; stay neutral and curious. **Then, take a few minutes to imagine what it would feel like if you had already achieved the health and wellness you desire.**

2. Complete the Uncover Your True *Wellness Why* worksheet.

Finding your *Wellness Why* may take time and iteration. Start with your initial gut reaction and continue to dig deeper with each iteration. **Use as many iterations as it takes to find it.** *Wellness Whys* elicit heartfelt and visceral feelings and emotions and are the true reason you want to achieve health and wellness, not surface reasons others impose on you, things you have to lose, or what is accepted in society and the media.

NOTE: Use the form in the guide or download the fillable PDF form for this activity in the Week 1 section on the book resource website.

3. Complete the Courage & Confidence Check.

It takes **courage** and **confidence** to let down your guard and emotionally go where you need to go to uncover your true *Wellness Why*. Did you muster the **courage** to go there? Are you **confident** you dug deep enough to uncover yours? How many iterations did it take for you to find it? The process of uncovering your true *Wellness Why* may raise strong thoughts, feelings, and fears that have been hidden deep inside you or that you have been avoiding.

a. **While uncovering my true *Wellness Why*, the thoughts and feelings I experienced were:**

_____

_____

b. Using a scale of 1-10 (with 10 being Extremely Confident and 1 being Not Very Confident At All), how **confident** are you that **you have found your true *Wellness Why?***

My current **confidence** level is:

1   2   3   4   5   6   7   8   9   10

What influenced my rating choice?

_____

_____

If my rating is less than 7, I may have not yet found my true *Wellness Why*, what can I do to increase my **confidence** that I will find it?

_____

_____

c. Feeling **confident** you were able to display the **courage** to find your true *Wellness Why* affects your **readiness to commit** to making changes. If your why is not compelling enough, you may not have moved the readiness needle much further.

Using a scale of 1-10 (with 10 being Extremely Ready and 1 being Not Being Ready at all), how has taking time to uncover your true *Wellness Why* affected your readiness to give yourself the gift of wellness?

My current **readiness** level is:

1   2   3   4   5   6   7   8   9   10

What influenced my rating choice?

_____

_____

If my rating is less than 7, what can I do to increase the **impact of my true *Wellness Why* on my readiness** to begin my journey toward my best self?

_____

_____

UNCOVER YOUR TRUE WELLNESS WHY WORKSHEET

Iteration #1 Why do I desire to give myself the gift of wellness now? I desire to:

Iteration #2 Why do I desire what I entered in Iteration #1? I desire to:

Iteration #3 Why do I desire what I entered in Iteration #2? I desire to:

Iteration #4 Why do I desire what I entered in Iteration #3? I desire to:

Iteration #5 Why do I desire what I entered in Iteration #4? I desire to:

Review all your iterations. Document your true Wellness Why? It may be a compilation of your iterations.
I desire to give myself the gift of wellness because:

NOTES & QUESTIONS TO BE ANSWERED

WEEK 2

SHOW UP & OWN IT

By showing up for yourself, you get to live, not simply exist.

"I continue to be amazed by our bodies' ability for self-repair. Our bodies want to be healthy if we would just let them."

–DR. MICHAEL GREGER

Did you know that everything you do in your life is because you want to feel something or believe you will feel something, but everything you resist doing is because you are avoiding feeling something or what you believe you will feel?

When you love to do something, you do it because it taps into your strengths. It's fun and engaging, and it keeps you motivated. This is what wellness authenticity feels like when you get there. Finding new health behaviors that feel this way takes time, but you will discover wellness authenticity using persistence and practice.

When you leverage your strengths to act authentically, courageously, and confidently, **you act as if you believe it is possible first** based on your beliefs about the future. When this happens, you will have the courage and confidence to take the next steps in your health and wellness journey.

In **Week 2**, you get to explore how your **innate strengths** support you stepping into your authentic wellness, and you get to believe, feel, and **act as if** you have already achieved the health and wellness you desire for life.

| 4 |

You Have What It Takes – Your Wellness Authenticity

Craft your own brand and flavor of health & wellness

Y ou already have what it takes to achieve your best self. Your values guide your work, and you use your strengths to be successful at work. **So why not leverage them to achieve your desired wellness?**

When you believe that what you are doing aligns with your strengths and values, you develop more positive thoughts, which leads to positive feelings about engaging in that activity and increases your motivation to do so. As a result, you are more likely to keep the activity at the top of your priority list.

It is a matter of rediscovering your strengths and being mindful about applying them to achieve the health and wellness you desire.

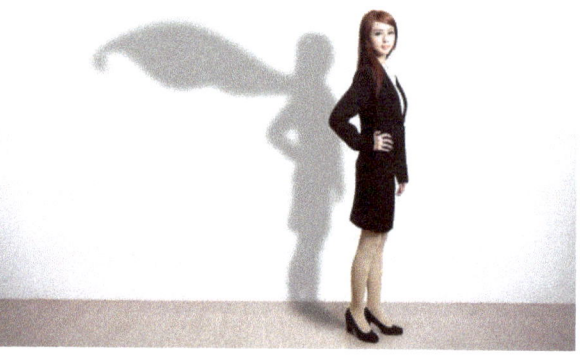

Use your strengths to craft your brand of health and wellness!

How can you use your identified strengths to help you be successful? By stepping back and examining your strengths from a different perspective, you will be amazed by what you learn about yourself.

Strategic Wellness Activities

It's time to leverage your innate strengths and abilities. You already have what it takes to create the positive, enthusiastic perspective necessary to achieve the health and wellness you desire.

1. Assess your current strengths and values.

Use the findings from a previous assessment or if you have not yet completed one or would like a refresher, try one of the suggested assessments.

> NOTE: The links to all strengths assessments are included in the Week 2 section on the book resource website.

a. **VIA Survey of Character Strengths** (Free) https://www.authentichappiness.sas.upenn.edu/user/login?destination=node/422
b. **High5Test** (Free) https://high5test.com/test/
c. **Top 5 Clifton Strengths** (Cost $19.99) https://www.gallup.com/cliftonstrengths/en/253868/popular-cliftonstrengths-assessment-products.aspx

2. Complete the *Wellness Authenticity* worksheet.

Identify how you get to leverage your top strengths and values to support your health and wellness journey.

a. **Enter your *Wellness Why* at the top of the worksheet.**
b. **List your top five strengths.**
c. **Describe what makes each important to you.**
d. **Identify situations in which you tend to use each strength the most.**
e. **Identify how you can leverage each strength to support your strategic wellness journey.**

> NOTE: Use the worksheet in the guide or download the full-size PDF fillable worksheet in the Week 2 section on the book resource website.

WELLNESS AUTHENTICITY WORKSHEET

a. My Wellness Why:

b. My Strengths	c. What makes this strength important to me?	d. In what situations do I tend to use this strength the most?	e. I will leverage this strength to support my Wellness Why and my strategic wellness journey by:

NOTES & QUESTIONS TO BE ANSWERED

| 5 |

Finding & Strengthening Your Wellness Presence

You get to think your way toward the wellness you desire!

Developing your *Wellness Presence* helps you give yourself permission to **take care of yourself first** and helps you use your new way of thinking and your strengths to build **readiness**, **importance**, **confidence**, and **excitement** about your ability to achieve and sustain the wellness you envision for yourself.

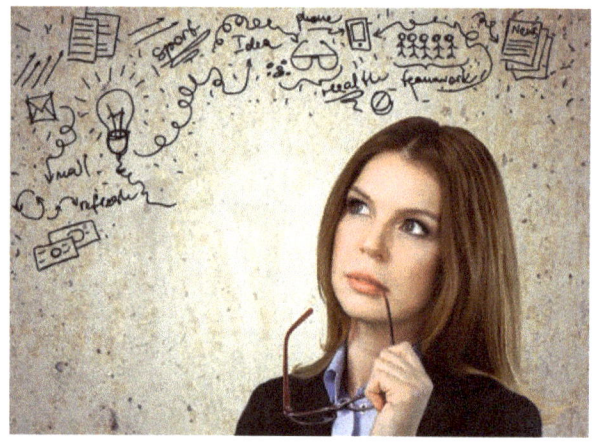

The only things holding you back are you and your brain!

It's time to realize and accept that there will always be someone and something holding you back from taking care of yourself. And hope is not a strategy!

The good news is: that someone holding you back is you and that something is your brain! You have total control over both using your superpower: your *Wellness Presence*. **Decide and own it!** Progress and mindset shift takes practice. Build your *Wellness Presence* every day!

Strategic Wellness Activities

Building your *Wellness Presence* to change your beliefs and thinking takes time. The strategic wellness activities help you become aware of your daily thoughts that you automatically accept as facts. You get to change them using your *Wellness Presence* building activities. Your beliefs and thoughts guide your associated behaviors; therefore, changing your beliefs and thoughts will change your behaviors.

1. Complete the *My Wellness Presence Building* worksheet.

The worksheet consists of four activities that build upon each other to help you first change your thinking by recognizing and reframing limiting thoughts. Then you create new thoughts and act on your new thinking to build new beliefs which elevate your readiness, importance, confidence, and enthusiasm related to your health and wellness journey. **Complete the entire sequence to begin building and sustaining your *Wellness Presence*.**

> NOTE: Use the worksheet in the guide or download the full-size PDF fillable worksheet in the Week 2 section on the book resource website.

Activity 1. Complete the **My RICE Analysis** to practice the process of changing your thinking by choosing your new thoughts about your levels of Readiness, Importance, Confidence, and Enthusiasm related to achieving the health and wellness you desire.

  a. In **Column a**, enter your current rating level for each RICE component from 1-10 (1 = Low to 10 = High).
  b. In **Column b**, for each component, identify the LIMITING thoughts and feelings you have that get in the way. Focus on the RICE component ratings less than 7; however, even if your rating is 7 or above, think of a limiting thought/feeling you've had that may have the potential to get in the way in the future. Also note where the limiting thought is coming from and what is the root cause.
  c. In **Column c**, decide if the limiting thought or feeling you are experiencing is a **Fact** or **Thought**. Facts are set in stone and would hold up in a court of law. Thoughts are simply sentences we repeat in our head, and we have the power to change them.
  d. In **Column d**, retire your old limiting thought and choose another thought from the "thought buffet" instead. What do you want this new perspective to mean to you?

Activity 2. Practice giving yourself permission to act on your new thought and translate it into action. This is when you truly begin building your *Wellness Presence*.

  a. **Every morning, look at yourself in the mirror and give yourself permission (out loud or silently) to take care of yourself.** The worksheet includes suggestions for key phrases to use when you see your reflection. Experiment with the phrases that work best for you.
  b. **Focus on the area of your RICE that feels off that week.** Feel free to practice your mirror activity when you need a lift throughout the day.

   c. **Act on your new thoughts** throughout the day (see Activity 3).

Activity 3. Think about a small daily action that aligns with your mirror conversation and brings your NEW thought to life.

   a. **Ask yourself**, "What would somebody with this new thought do to achieve their best self?"

   b. **Then, act "as if."** Choose at least one small daily action that aligns with your strengths and values; feel free to do more. The worksheet contains suggestions. Always do what feels authentic for you.

Activity 4. Spend 5-10 minutes reflecting every evening or first thing in the morning on how you did with your Wellness Presence building process.

   a. Enter the new thoughts on which you acted.

   b. Enter the mirror phrases you used.

   c. Enter the action(s) you took that day to live your thought.

   d. Note what felt most effective for you and what you want to continue doing. What phrases or sentences energized you? What activities felt right for you? Reflect on the phrases that gave you the power to act on your thoughts and the actions that felt more natural for you and aligned with your strengths.

Sustaining your *Wellness Presence* by leveraging your strengths and values and staying aligned with your true *Wellness Why* is an effective tactic to help get you started and continue to smooth over the bumps in the road along your wellness journey.

Eventually, you will feel your *Wellness Presence* and see it in yourself. Others will see it, too, and may comment on the changes they see. However, until you genuinely think it and feel it, you may feel like a fraud or as if you are going through the motions. Don't give up. You will struggle with achieving and sustaining your health and wellness until you find and believe in your *Wellness Presence*. You must show up for yourself on the inside first and lead your journey!

2. Complete the Courage & Confidence Check.

What are your thoughts and feelings about performing the activities to build your *Wellness Presence*? It may feel stupid, unnatural, or anxiety-provoking for you – resist these feelings, and don't give in! Can you **commit** to evaluating your *Wellness Presence* daily and taking action to build it?

It takes **courage** and **confidence** to step out of your comfort zone every day to build your *Wellness Presence.*

Using a scale of 1-10 (with 10 being Extremely Committed and 1 being Not Very Committed At All), how **committed** are you to take daily action to build the *Wellness Presence* you need to support the achievement of the health and wellness you desire?

My **commitment** level is:

1   2   3   4   5   6   7   8   9   10

What influenced my rating choice?

_____

_____

If my rating is less than 7, what can I do to increase my **commitment** level to perform daily actions to build my *Wellness Presence?*

_____

_____

WELLNESS PRESENCE BUILDING WORKSHEET

Activity #1: Build Your RICE by Changing Your Thinking

You control your thoughts. Your thoughts directly affect the components of your RICE. Think about how you feel about giving yourself the gift of wellness now. For each component, rate your level using a scale of 1-10 (with 1 = low and 10 = high). Next, identify your limiting thoughts that are getting in the way and choose a better/new thought. Think about what you want this new perspective to mean to you.

Component	a. Rating (1-10)	b. What are the limiting thoughts and feelings that are getting in my way? Where are these coming from?	c. Fact or Thought?	d. I choose this new thought/belief instead. What do I want this new perspective to mean?
Readiness				
Importance (Priority)				
Confidence				
Enthusiasm				

WELLNESS PRESENCE BUILDING WORKSHEET, cont.

Activity #2: Exercise Your Wellness Presence – Give Yourself Permission to Act on Your New Thought/Belief

It's time for you to start taking care of YOU! If you are not feeling well, how can you be your best self when taking care of others at home and supporting your people at work? Every morning, look at yourself in the mirror and give yourself permission (out loud or silently) to take care of yourself and exercise your new thoughts/beliefs so you can be your best self. Feel free to practice throughout the day when you need a lift. Use the suggestions below or make up your own.

"I deserve the gift of health and wellness."	"Be, don't try to become."	
"I am NOT at the mercy of my genetics."	"I choose to treat my health as an important wealth."	
"I am ready to live well and lead well."	"I am open to receiving the gift of health now."	"I am confident I can make a change now."

Activity #3: Be and Do – Align Your Actions With Your New Thoughts

What would someone who has already achieved their best self do? Choose one of the short actions from the list below (or make up your own) to perform daily to build and sustain your new thoughts/beliefs about your Readiness, Importance, Confidence, and Enthusiasm to demonstrate your commitment to giving yourself the gift of wellness.

- Smile for 30 seconds
- Laugh about something funny that happened to you today
- Drink 1 extra glass of water
- Recognize someone for great work
- Stay positive when speaking to others
- Stand up and stretch
- Avoid alcohol within 3 hours of bedtime
- Do 5 squats at your desk
- Take 5 minutes and do a future pull

- Pack and eat a fruit snack
- Do heel lifts when waiting for your tea or coffee to brew
- Skip a snack in the breakroom
- Eat one meal without meat, eggs, or dairy
- Stop eating 3 hours before bedtime
- Walk outside for 5 minutes
- Schedule a fun event with a friend
- Go home from work on time
- Meditate for 5 minutes before bedtime

- Listen to your favorite song
- Before you go in the house after work, walk around the block for 5 minutes.
- Walk while talking on the phone
- Think of one thing for which you are grateful
- Skip the afternoon caffeine and go for a walk instead
- Use the stairs between meetings
- Be flexible to accommodate others
- Be there for someone in need
- Close your eyes and take 5 slow deep breaths

Activity #4: Wellness Presence Building Reflection

At first, it may be helpful to reflect in the evening about how you did with choosing your new thoughts. This is often difficult for people to do. Make a note of the phrases that gave you the feelings you needed to take action on your thoughts and which actions felt more natural for you aligned with your strengths.

Daily Reflection Format

Date	The new thought/belief I acted on today was:	The mirror statement I told myself to incite my feelings and desire to act were:	The small action I took to live my new thought was:	How did I feel taking action? What will I continue to do tomorrow? What will I change? Other thoughts?

NOTES & QUESTIONS TO BE ANSWERED

WEEK 3

FORMULATING YOUR NEW BELIEFS

Until you learn how to reprogram your subconscious, you will not change a thing. Embrace who you get to be, not who you've been!

"There's nothing more important than our good health – that's our principal capital asset."

—ARLEN SPECTER

One of my favorite quotes I use in my writing and speaking is, *"I want to die from a chronic disease I could have prevented,"* said no one ever! But, according to the American College of Lifestyle Medicine, **80 percent of premature deaths are attributable to poor diet, physical inactivity, and tobacco** use, and **78 percent of patients seen in primary care have lifestyle-related conditions**.

So based on these statistics, people are speaking this quote with their actions. They may consciously verbalize they *want to be healthy and live a long life*, but actions speak louder than words and do not lie. **They do as they do, not as they say. I believe people mean well, and I believe they do want to live a healthy life.** The disconnect happens in the brain because your conscious brain only controls 5 percent of your thinking. Your subconscious brain expresses your beliefs about what's possible for you and the actions you take. The subconscious part of your brain is in control 95 percent of the time.

Creating your *Lifestyle Wellness Strategic Plan* helps you shift to leveraging this powerful 95 percent of your brain to support your health and wellness. The power is inside you - manage your mind and create your own experiences.

In **Week 3**, you continue building a solid foundation upon which to **develop new beliefs** and finally get unstuck, move forward, and **embrace new possibilities**.

| 6 |

What Do You Have to Gain?

If you say it but you doubt it, nothing changes.

We all tend to struggle with change. **It's important to understand that this is normal, and don't be surprised when it occurs.** You can be sure you will sometimes struggle when making health and wellness changes and will often fall off the wagon.

When it happens, "Go With It," and don't get discouraged...**give yourself time to adapt and work through the unknowns and challenges**. It takes time for your conscious brain to be in charge. Until then, your old, automatic thoughts that no longer serve you try to emerge and take over.

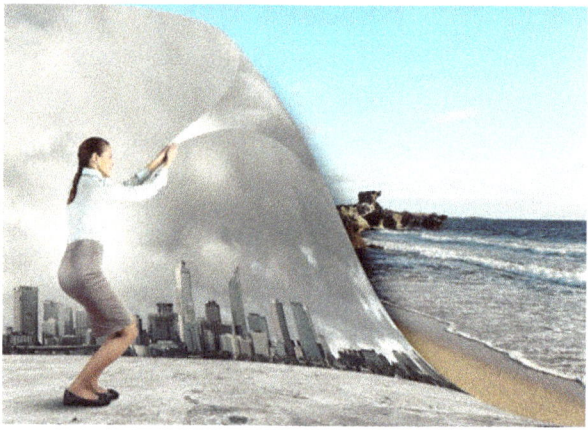

Only you can change your life by changing your thinking first.

Stay strong and use the activities in this chapter and the next to work through the feelings and challenges. **If you give up too soon, you will risk losing the chance to be creative and develop into what you need to renew yourself.**

Strategic Wellness Activities

The strategic wellness planning process is your transition phase; however, the duration of your transition phase is unique to you. Transitioning allows time to shift your mindset and develop a clearer picture of what changes you get to make to be the best version of yourself - BEFORE you make the changes.

1. Complete the reflective writing activity.

Think about a time when you used a positive approach to change.

a. Describe a change that you consider a high point or peak experience in your life or work.

_____

_____

_____

b. What thoughts did you have about making this change? How did these thoughts about the change make you feel? What did you GAIN from making the change?

_____

_____

_____

c. How did you prepare yourself for making this change?

_____

_____

_____

d. What helped you stick with the change after you made it?

_____

_____

_____

e. How did your people and support systems help you build a strong foundation for making the change?

_____

_____

_____

f. How can you leverage the positive approach to transition you described above to achieve your health and wellness goals by focusing on what you will GAIN?

_____

_____

_____

2. Complete the reflective writing activity.

Now think about a change or situation you feel did not go so well for you. Take a moment to reframe and reimagine this change as a high point in your life.

a. Describe a change that you believe did not go so well for you.

_____

_____

_____

b. How could you change your thinking and reframe the situation from a positive transition perspective?

_____

_____

_____

c. How have you become a better person or moved forward from the change?

_____

_____

_____

3. Complete the Courage & Confidence Check.

If you are looking for someone to change your life, look in the mirror! Only you can change your life by changing your thinking first before your actions.

a. **What are your thoughts and feelings about knowing you will have to make some changes in your life to achieve the health and wellness you desire**? Do you have the courage to take the steps to create the conditions for a positive transition? Which of the following describes you?

I will have the **courage** to create the conditions for a positive transition:

_____ Not for a while   _____ In about 6 months

_____ In about 3 months   _____ Within 1 month

_____ Already taking action

b. Using a scale of 1-10 (with 10 being Extremely Confident and 1 being Not Very Confident At All), how **confident** are you in your ability to effectively transition before making changes and view the changes in a positive light--as something you gain versus lose--when you initiate your transition?

My **confidence** level is:

1   2   3   4   5   6   7   8   9   10

What influenced my rating choice?

_____

_____

If my rating is less than 7, I will take the following actions to increase my **confidence** level to effectively create a positive transition:

_____

_____

NOTES & QUESTIONS TO BE ANSWERED

| 7 |

What Do You Have to Lose?

When you embrace who you really are and what is, you'll change.

Before you can begin something new, you must end what used to be. **Before you can learn a new way of doing things, you must unlearn the old ways.** Before you can become a different kind of person, you must let go of your old identity.

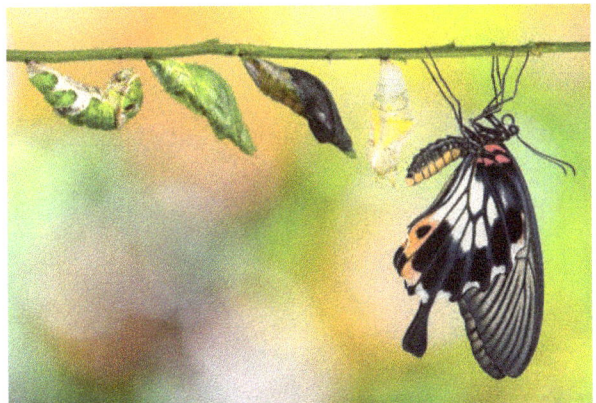

Begin creating the new thoughts that will transform your health and wellness.

Habits are ingrained and serve a purpose. **It's time to recognize the old habits that no longer support your health and wellness and put them to rest.** They were there when you needed them, but it's now time to have them rest in peace. Your current habits and routines are part of your current reality and impact who you are and who you have been.

Accept that fact, and **don't be surprised if you feel angry, sad, passionate, or adamant about giving up something that you feel has given you pleasure, comfort, relaxation, or escape**. A piece of your world is being lost. You must purge and manage any negative thoughts and feelings getting in the way of achieving your desired health and wellness.

Strategic Wellness Activities

You know you will need to permanently give up and reduce the frequency of unhealthy behaviors *enough* to achieve the wellness you desire--again, don't believe anyone who tells you otherwise. Before you flip the change switch, let's continue the positive psychological transition so you can manage and put the associated negative thoughts and emotions to rest. It takes time and deliberate effort to permanently make healthy lifestyle choices superior to unhealthy default habits and choices. You must call upon what you've learned about yourself thus far.

1. Complete the *Losing → Gaining Postive Transition* worksheet.

This activity will help you actively create new positive thoughts about what you will gain by giving up or managing the habits, behaviors, thoughts, and concerns that you feel are getting in the way of your ability to give yourself the gift of wellness now.

> NOTE: Use the worksheet in the guide or download the full-size PDF fillable worksheet in the Week 3 section on the book resource website.

a. Enter your *Wellness Why*.
b. Then list 1-3 habits, behaviors, or thoughts you feel you will struggle with the most while achieving your desired health and wellness.
c. Next, determine if these align with your true *Wellness Why*.
d. Determine what you will have to give up for each item on your list and how you feel about it.
e. Shift your thinking to focus on what you will gain from eliminating the habit or behavior, and then select a new wellness activity you can do instead or when you feel triggered. Choose activities and distractions that align with your strengths and values.
f. Finally, identify how you will "mourn" giving up this habit or behavior using your *Wellness Presence* building process. This step is a way for you to accept and validate the thoughts and feelings you are experiencing and what you can do to "mourn the loss" of a longstanding, comfortable place so you can completely alleviate or shift your thoughts and feelings.

2. Complete the Courage & Confidence Check.

Understanding how to create conditions to make a positive psychological transition before you make changes is the only way you will make wellness feel natural to you and make the healthy choice the easier choice. As your life and career unfold, you will need to call upon these skills to adapt to changes and challenges in other areas.

As your wellness improves and you become more **courageous** and **confident**, you will want to do more. But don't let your guard down--don't think you can do more without going through the positive transition process. Along your wellness journey, loss is loss. Regardless of where you are and how long you've been on your journey, you must accept, grieve, and move forward toward a positive future.

a. Using a scale of 1-10 (with 10 being Extremely Confident and 1 being Not Very Confident At All), how **confident** are you in your ability to effectively accept, mourn, and let go or give up old habits, behaviors, thoughts, and concerns when you decide to begin your wellness journey?

My **confidence** level is:

1   2   3   4   5   6   7   8   9   10

What influenced my rating choice?

_____

_____

If my rating is less than 7, I will take the following actions to increase my **confidence** level to effectively put my unhealthy habits, behaviors, and concerns to rest:

_____

_____

b. Using a scale of 1-10 (with 10 being Extremely Courageous and 1 being Not Very Courageous At All), how **courageous** do you feel in your ability to wrangle with the uncomfortable thoughts and feelings that go along with the psychological transition when giving up old habits and behaviors, ?

My **courage** level is:

1   2   3   4   5   6   7   8   9   10

What influenced my rating choice?

_____

_____

If my rating is less than 7, I will take the following actions to increase my **courage** level to manage my positive transition:

_____

_____

LOSING-->GAINING TRANSITION WORKSHEET

You know you will need to permanently give up and reduce the frequency of unhealthy behaviors ENOUGH to achieve the wellness you desire. You must manage and put to rest the associated negative thoughts and emotions to facilitate a positive, psychological transition before you make the change. It takes time and deliberate effort to permanently make healthy lifestyle choices superior to unhealthy default habits.

a. My True Wellness Why: _____

b. What habits, behaviors, concerns, thoughts, or feelings affect my ability to give myself the gift of wellness?	c. Does this behavior align with my true Wellness Why? (Yes/No)	d. What habit or behavior will I have to give up, eliminating this habit or behavior? How do I feel about this?	e. What will I gain from managing or eliminating this habit or behavior? What will be my new way of thinking about this?	f. What positive distraction or healthy replacement activity can I do instead? (Identify a distraction aligned with your strengths. Who can support you?)	g. How will I mourn the loss of this habit/behavior? (Use your Wellness Presence building to mourn this habit, shift your thinking and lay it to rest for good.)
1.					
2.					
3.					

NOTES & QUESTIONS TO BE ANSWERED

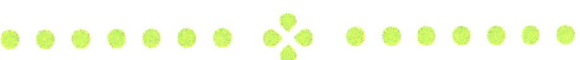

WEEK 4

ENDLESS POSSIBILITIES ARE YOURS

Believe your way to the health and wellness you desire.

"You can't change life at the action level, but you can by using the domino effect: Changed thoughts/beliefs-->change feelings--> change actions-->change results."

-LIZ NICKLAS

Most people are trying to change reality first; however, **you must first work on the believing, and then the reality will catch up with what you believe.**

Your reality is being constructed by how you think. Your thoughts create your evidence. Beliefs are thoughts you think over and over. They are programs running in all areas of your brain. You expect things to work out a certain way based on your beliefs. Beliefs create expectations, and those expectations create your life. Your life is what you expect to find. Your practiced beliefs are expectations, and your expectations have creative power.

Reality is fixed, but your *personal reality* is not; it is your interpretation. Interestingly, your subconscious does not know the difference between reality and future vision. You tell it what to believe by transforming the vision of your identity. It's time to create the health and wellness beliefs that create the expectations for the future vision you get to have.

In **Week 4**, you get to **envision your wellness future** and what you want to see and experience along the way. Have fun and **experience the joy** of having endless possibilities.

| 8 |

Visualize Your Future Direction

Think ahead of where you are. Create it and then practice believing it.

If you feel life is always the same, then it is because you are recycling old thoughts. This could be a good thing or a bad thing. When things in your life feel in order and routine, this breeds habit and makes it hard to change, especially related to your health and wellness.

Comfort builds complacency: however, **chaos often breeds life**. You know you need to make changes; however, you may feel disorganized or unsure where to start.

These feelings make people jump into action quickly, doing the same things that may not have worked in the past. They make New Year's resolutions that don't stick, such as joining a gym, cutting carbs, or quitting something *cold turkey* (or cold tofu).

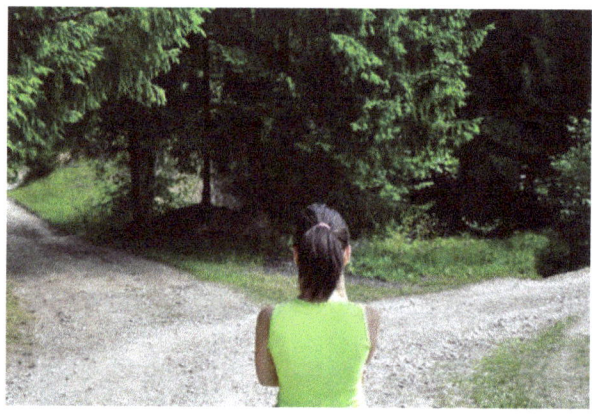
Are you ready to choose the road less traveled?

Everything you believe about your health and wellness comes from something you already believe. **When you think ahead of where you are, you create new beliefs from the future**--choose what you want to believe, think, and act to create your future direction.

Strategic Wellness Activities

You get to imagine what stepping out of your health and wellness reality would look like. Your current reality does not have to define your future unless you let it. By examining the pros and cons for changing and for staying the same, you begin to experience what believing ahead of where

52

you are feels like. It often provides an uncomfortable dose of reality. It's time to change that and take a dose of new beliefs daily.

1. Complete the *Choose Your Future Direction* worksheet.

Plan 15-20 minutes of quiet, uninterrupted time to complete this activity. Think about your true *Wellness Why*, and where you are now. Compare and contrast how it would look to stay the same or change your reality by changing what you believe.

> NOTE: Use the form in the guide or download the full-size PDF fillable worksheet in the Week 4 section on the book resource website.

   a. List the pros for staying the same.
   b. List the cons for staying the same.
   c. List the pros for making changes to give yourself the gift of wellness
   d. List the cons for making changes to give yourself the gift of wellness.
   e. Based on the items on your list, develop a creative name for your Stay the Same road.
   f. Based on the items on your list, develop a creative name for your Make the Change road.
   g. Choose the road you want to take and post the name of the road on your wall as a reminder about where you want to go.
   h. Reflect on your road choice.

2. Complete the reflective writing activity.

Can you commit to traveling down the road to change? Open your curious mind to all the incredible new possibilities to come! Think about a recent vacation or trip you enjoyed. You most likely had a plan and did what you could to ensure you had a positive, engaging time. Before your venture, you most likely crafted a positive visualization of your experience in your mind's eye and kept your visualization at the forefront of your thinking.

The same is true for your health and wellness journey. As you imagined yourself standing at the fork, could you feel and create a positive vision of what it would be like along the road to change? The more pros for changing, the greater your motivation to leave your default reality behind.

   a. **What thoughts and feelings are you having about choosing the road to change?**

   _____
   _____
   _____

   b. **What is holding you back? How can you change your perspective to prepare to take the road less travelled?**

_____

_____

_____

_____

3. Complete the Courage & Confidence Check.

Choosing the road to change takes **courage** and **confidence**–both boosted by taking time to create the conditions to make a positive psychological transition before you make the change.

a. Do you have the **courage** and **confidence** to take the first steps down your road to change? Is the image of your positive health and wellness future drawing you forward? The first steps to getting started are sometimes the hardest to take. Having a positive visual may make it easier.

Using a scale of 1-10 (with 10 being Extremely Courageous and 1 being Not Very Courageous At All), how **courageous** do you feel about taking the first steps down the positive road to change you have visualized to achieve a positive transition?

My **courage** level is:

1   2   3   4   5   6   7   8   9   10

What influenced my rating choice?

_____

_____

If my rating is less than 7, I will take the following actions to increase my **courage** level to take the first steps down the positive road to change:

_____

_____

b. Your true _Wellness Why_, combined with your positive visualization down the road to change, are significant inputs into building the **confidence** that you can achieve and sustain the wellness you desire. You see the choices you have and the implications each choice has on your health and wellness future.

Using a scale of 1-10 (with 10 being Extremely Confident and 1 being Not Very Confident At All), how **confident** are you in taking the next steps down the road to change and keep it going in the long term?

My **confidence** level is:

1   2   3   4   5   6   7   8   9   10

What influenced my rating choice?

_____

_____

If my rating is less than 7, I will take the following actions to increase my **confidence** level to take the next steps down the road to change and keep it going:

_____

_____

CHOOSE YOUR FUTURE DIRECTION

Think about your true "Wellness Why" and where you are now.
- On the left side, list the Pros and Cons for Staying the Same.
- On the right side, list the Pros and Cons for Making the Change.
- After you have completed your lists, create a name for each road which serves as a metaphor about where you will end up if you choose to take each fork.

YOUR HEALTH & WELLNESS FORK IN THE ROAD

a. Staying the Same - Pros   **c. Making the Change - Pros**

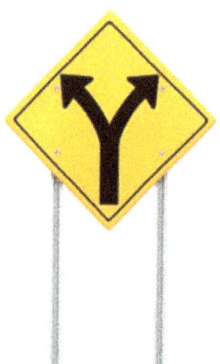

b. Staying the Same - Cons   **d. Making the Change - Cons**

e. "Staying the Same" Road Name: **f. "Making the Change" Road Name:**

g. Which health and wellness fork do you get to take?

h. What are your thoughts and feelings about the fork you chose?

NOTES & QUESTIONS TO BE ANSWERED

| 9 |

The Reality of the Future You

Believing puts the future you right in front of you; step into your authentic wellness.

Your wellness journey isn't simply crossing from one side of the street to the other. **It's a journey of a lifetime, from one identity to another, which takes time.**

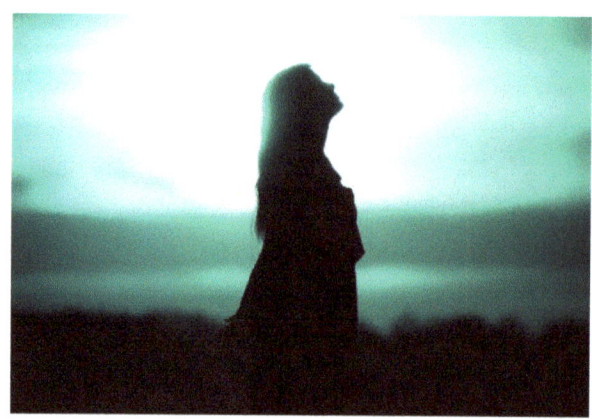

Your Wellness Vision brings your wellness journey to life - Your Life!

I'm confident you've decided to take the road to change. The next step is deciding how your journey will look as you move forward. This is your *Wellness Vision*. It is what you see and feel when you think of living your best self.

Your *Wellness Vision* should feel like a stretch for you, yet attainable. It is future-oriented but created in the present tense using "I am" statements.

Your *Wellness Vision* is driven by your *Wellness Why* and accentuates the **pros** you identified for choosing your road to change. You may not yet have a clear *Wellness Vision*. However, I guarantee you will by the time you complete your *Lifestyle Wellness Strategic Plan*.

Strategic Wellness Activities

Again, it's time to relax, get creative, and open your mind to visualizing the infinite possibilities of your best self! You will use your list of **pros for choosing the road to wellness** as an input to create your official *Wellness Vision* aligned with your *Wellness Why* and keep it authentic by aligning it with your strengths and values. Your *Wellness Vision* will serve as your beacon throughout your wellness journey.

Set aside 15 minutes of quiet, uninterrupted time to complete this activity. Relax, close your eyes, take a deep breath, and picture yourself in your desired future. How do you look? What are you doing? How are you feeling? Who are you with? Take the time you need to visualize your future self fully.

1. Complete the *Create Your Wellness Vision* worksheet.

Create your future-oriented *Wellness Vision* using "I" and "I am" statements as if in the present tense. Your *Wellness Vision* is driven by your *Wellness Why*, aligned with your strengths, and accentuates the pros for changing.

> **NOTE: Use the form in the guide or download the full-size PDF fillable worksheet in the Week 4 section on the book resource website.**

    a. Enter your *Wellness Why*.
    b. Enter your top 5 strengths.
    c. Review your list of pros you created for choosing the road to change. Complete the column labeled **Values & Desires**. Ask yourself, what do I desire as a positive future outcome? What is most important to me?
    d. Next, complete the column labeled **Actions**. Ask yourself, what needs to happen for me to realize each desire and live my values?
    e. Combine and summarize all your actions with the associated values & desires to create your *Wellness Vision* using the formula "I am (action) so I (realizing my desires and living my values)" It may take a few iterations, but you will get there. Review the examples in the book to assist you.

2. Complete the Courage & Confidence Check.

Your *Wellness Vision* contributes to the motivational energy that will move you forward through the change process. It considers your best experiences, core strengths and values, and support systems to help you imagine the way forward.

    a. Your clear *Wellness Vision* gives you the **confidence** to move forward toward your health and wellness target. Your confidence will continue to grow along the way.

    Using a scale of 1-10 (with 10 being Extremely Confident and 1 being Not Very Confident At All), how **confident** do you feel that you have created a compelling *Wellness Vision* that will keep you moving forward in your wellness journey?

My **confidence** level is:

1   2   3   4   5   6   7   8   9   10

What influenced my rating choice?

_____

_____

If my rating was is than 7, I will take the following actions to increase my **confidence** in my *Wellness Vision* to keep moving forward:

_____

_____

b. Your *Wellness Vision* creates a visual in your mind's eye to help you stay positive and focused throughout your wellness journey. A clear vision gives you the courage to willingly embark on your wellness journey – you can see what the future will be.

Using a scale of 1-10 (with 10 being Extremely Courageous and 1 being Not Very Courageous At All), how **courageous** are you feeling to face your wellness future and live your *Wellness Vision*?

My **courage** level is:

1   2   3   4   5   6   7   8   9   10

What influenced my rating choice?

_____

_____

If my rating is less than 7, I will take the following actions to increase my **courage** level to take the next steps to face my wellness future and live my vision:

_____

_____

CREATE YOUR WELLNESS VISION

Think about what life looks like and feels like when you get to be your best self.

a. My Wellness Why:

b. My Top 5 Strengths to Leverage:

c. Being (I AM)	d. Values & Desires (SO THAT)
Sample: I am eating mindfully	*so I can enjoy food while reducing my risk of heart attack.*
1.	
2.	
3.	
4.	
5.	
6.	
7.	
8.	

e. My Wellness Vision

I am (being) so that I (realize my desires and live my values)

NOTES & QUESTIONS TO BE ANSWERED

WEEK 5

MEET YOUR FUTURE SELF NOW

Your future self is within your control.

"Even after years of beating yourself up with a horrible diet, your body can reverse the damage, open back up the arteries-even reverse the progression of some cancers. Amazing! So, it's never too late to start exercising, never too late to stop smoking, never too late to get better sleep, and never too late to start eating healthier."

-DR. MICHAEL GREGER

Reality is not fixed; it is only your interpretation. Your life right now is the effect of what you believe is possible, and nothing can change until you learn to change your subconscious beliefs.

Your current health and wellness reality reflects your current beliefs and thinking, which keep you stuck and create behavior patterns that are no longer serving you.

When you truly believe in something, that is when you can create it. Build certainty into your life around the goals and dreams you have. Certainty is believing you are the person already! And then reality catches up with you. Most people are trying to change reality first; you get to work on the believing so reality will catch up with what you believe.

In **Week 5**, you get to candidly evaluate **your current health and wellness reality**, determine if you like where you are, and then decide **how willing you are and how much you want to invest** in experiencing your *Wellness Vision*.

| 10 |

Your Current Reality

The good, the bad, the ugly! Your past does not equal your future!

You've been focusing on the psychological component of health and wellness. It's now time to shift to examining the physical component: **your current health behaviors and choices**. This makes up your current self (reality) and where you are right now with living a lifestyle of health and wellness.

Developing an awareness of your current reality and how you feel about it drive your motivation to change.

If you are okay with your current reality, you may be less likely to make any changes or the changes you do make won't stick. That's okay, however, I don't think that is the case. **I believe you are over the status quo.**

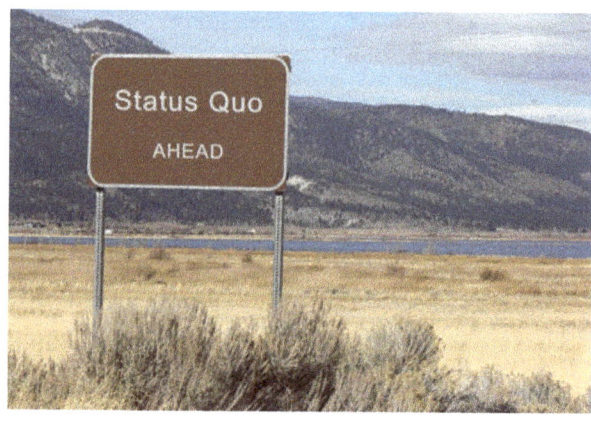

Don't be okay with your health and wellness status quo and more of the same?

If your current reality is not acceptable, then an evaluation is the first step to helping you decide how far you are willing to go to create your new reality, the new you that you envision.

Strategic Wellness Activities

This strategic wellness activity includes a self-evaluation to help you think about where you are for each **Lifestyle Wellness Component** and establish your *Current Baseline* for Nutrition, Movement, Sleep, Stress Management, Positivity & Meaningful Connections, Risky Substance Avoidance, and Supportive Home & Work Environments.

You will use my theoretical Chronic Diseases of Lifestyle Risk Progression Model to establish your *Current Baseline* **ratings.**

CHRONIC DISEASES OF LIFESTYE PROGRESSION MODEL

Less Healthy
Low Control/Willingness

Extremely Healthy
High Control/Willingness

Incite & Accelerate	Slow Progression	Mitigate & Arrest	Prevent & Reverse

10%	20	30	40	50%	60	70	80	90	100%

1. Download the *Current & Future Reality Self-Evaluation* **form and enter you** *Current Baseline* **ratings.**

Your *Current Baseline* for each of these components is the starting point for your journey. A journey always needs a starting point. You need to know where you are to get where you want to be. The roadmap for your journey will be personalized for you, depending on where you start and where you see your wellness future.

Your *Current & Future Reality Self-Evaluation* helps you gauge where you are with the components of your Lifestyle Wellness and guides your decisions about your future wellness target for each.

> NOTE: Download the fillable PDF evaluation form in the Week 5 section on the book resource website.

> a. Complete **only** the *Current Baseline* rating in cell a. for each component. **This is your perception of where you are for each lifestyle wellness component.** In the next chapter, you will complete your *Desired Goal* and *Willingness to Invest* ratings.

> **To complete your evaluation**, review the description for each *Lifestyle Wellness Component* and rate how the percentage of your current behaviors (*Current Baseline*) aligns with the description. Use the rating scale: 10% = Less Healthy/Low Control/Low Willingness to 100% = Extremely Healthy/High Control/High Willingness.

> **EXAMPLE:** In this example, the wellness investor rates her Nutrition *Current Baseline* at 20%. She rarely eats fruits and vegetables and often follows the ketogenic diet, by consuming ultra-processed meal replacement bars, deli meat, prepackaged snacks, and fast foods high in added fat, oil, and salt. In addition, she drinks 3-4 artificially sweetened beverages daily.

Less Healthy			Extremely Healthy
Low Control/Willingness			High Control/Willingness

Incite & Accelerate   Slow Progression   Mitigate & Arrest   Prevent & Reverse

10%   20   30   40   50%   60   70   80   90   100%

Nutrition - My nutritional plan is based predominately on a variety of minimally processed whole plant-based foods, limited meat and animal products, low added sugar, salt and oil, and high in fruits, vegetables, beans, legumes, and whole grains.

a) My Nutrition Current Baseline:	b) My Nutrition Desired Goal:	c) My Willingness to Invest to Achieve My Nutrition Desired Goal:	d) My Nutrition Future Target:
20			

Example: Current Baseline rating for Healthful Nutrition

2. Complete the Courage & Confidence Check.

Nobody likes giving or receiving a low rating on an evaluation. Low ratings may create discomfort, especially when you feel you have limited control over changing your health status. Fortunately, that's not always the case when using lifestyle medicine practices – it's never too late to make a difference. However, the longer you wait, the more damage you may be doing to your body, creating a greater risk that the damage is irreversible.

a. It takes **courage** and **confidence** to get real and face the current state of your health and wellness – no sugarcoating and no excuses.

Using a scale of 1-10 (with 10 being Extremely Courageous and 1 being Not Very Courageous At All), how **courageous** and **confident** were you to face the current state of your wellness?

My **courage** level is:

1   2   3   4   5   6   7   8   9   10

My **confidence** level is:

1   2   3   4   5   6   7   8   9   10

What influenced my rating choices?

_____

_____

If my ratings are less than 7, I will take the following actions to increase my **courage** and **confidence** levels to face the current state of my wellness:

_____

_____

NOTES & QUESTIONS TO BE ANSWERED

| 11 |

How Much Will You Invest?

Don't wait until you lose your health before you decide to value it! The first wealth is health!

Y ou are probably beginning to recognize that your old patterns and habits are not consistent with your *Wellness Vision,* and if you don't make changes, you will not experience what you see in your *Wellness Vision.*

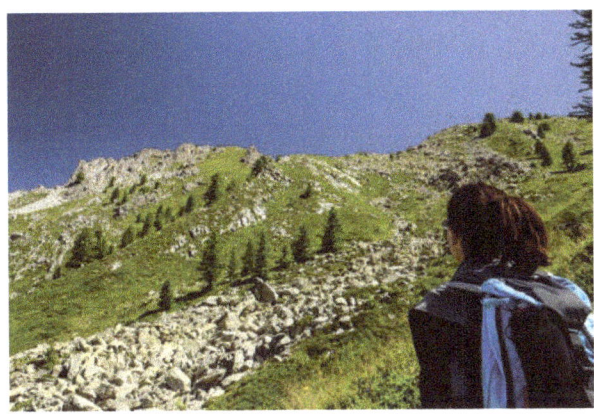

How willing are you to invest in achieving your desired goals?

Mindsets are self-fulfilling prophesies: If you think you can improve, you will. If you think you are stuck, you are. However, mindsets are learned and can be changed. A growth mindset thrives on challenge and sees failure not as evidence of incompetence or unintelligence but as a springboard for learning, growth, and stretching our existing abilities. Achieving your *Wellness Vision* is possible when you adopt a growth mindset.

When you are ready to implement your *Lifestyle Wellness Strategic Plan,* you will be encouraged to experiment with new ideas and embrace your successes and less than successes. **You never fail; you learn, adapt, and move forward.** So how far are you willing to go to give yourself the gift of wellness?

Strategic Wellness Activities

In the previous chapter's strategic wellness activity, you entered your *Current Baseline* ratings for each lifestyle wellness component. Next, it's time to think about what you want your future to look like and how willing you are to act on your new beliefs. When you believe ahead of where you are – your thoughts will create your future.

1. Use the Current & Future Reality Self-Evaluation form from the previous chapter to enter you *Desired Goal* and *Willingness to Invest* ratings.

Now that you've had time to reflect on your initial *Current Baseline* ratings, feel free to review and adjust them if necessary.

> NOTE: If you have not yet done so, download the full-size PDF fillable evaluation form in the Week 5 section on the book resource website.

a. Enter your **Desired Goal** for each component using the same 10-100% rating range. Your *Desired Goal* is essentially your authentic goal for each component. This is the level that aligns with achieving your *Wellness Vision* and that you choose to invest in and sustain throughout your lifelong wellness journey.

b. Next, enter your **Willingness to Invest** rating for each component. Your *Willingness to Invest* rating is how willing and likely you will make and sustain enough changes to achieve your *Desired Goal*.

c. Your **Future Target** ratings will be auto-calculated based on your *Current Baseline, Desired Goal*, and *Willingness to Invest* ratings.

d. Review your *Future Targets* for each component and your *Overall Lifestyle Wellness* calculations at the bottom of the second page. Your Overall Lifestyle Wellness rating fields are auto-calculated based on the average ratings of the other components.

2. Conduct a final review of all your self-ratings.

Do your ratings reflect your current self and desired future self. Be sure you feel good about your self-ratings and believe you've entered **candid** *Current Baselines*, **realistic** *Desired Goals*, and **confident** *Willingness to Invest* ratings.

> **EXAMPLE:** Continuing the example from the previous chapter, this wellness investor rated her **Nutrition Desired Goal at 60%.** Her *Wellness Vision* aligned with crafting her *Lifestyle Wellness Strategic Plan* to potentially *slow or stabilize the progression* of her chronic diseases of lifestyle. She felt **90% Willing and Confident to Invest** in working toward aligning her behaviors with 60% of the *Evidence-Based Quality Standard (EBQS).*
>
> She had active diseases managed by medication. Based on her *Desired Goal* and *Willingness to Invest* ratings, her **Future Target** calculated to **56%** of the EBQS, which aligns with her *Wellness Vision* of potentially slowing and stabilizing the progression of her chronic diseases of lifestyle. She said this Nutritional level felt doable and authentic for her lifestyle, and she may eventually decide to raise her *Future Target.*

Less Healthy
Low Control/Willingness

Extremely Healthy
High Control/Willingness

| Incite & Accelerate | Slow Progression | Mitigate & Arrest | Prevent & Reverse |

10%   20   30   40   50%   60   70   80   90   100%

Nutrition - My nutritional plan is based predominately on a variety of minimally processed whole plant-based foods, limited meat and animal products, low added sugar, salt and oil, and high in fruits, vegetables, beans, legumes, and whole grains.

a) My Nutrition Current Baseline:	b) My Nutrition Desired Goal:	c) My Willingness to Invest to Achieve My Nutrition Desired Goal:	d) My Nutrition Future Target:
20	60	90	56

Example: Desired Goal, Willingness to Invest, & Future Target ratings for Healthful Nutrition

Her *Overall Lifestyle Wellness* ratings present a composite average including ratings for all eight components. Her calculated *Overall Lifestyle Wellness Future Target* is 77% and also aligns with her *Wellness Vision.* These composite ratings are affected by higher *Current Baseline* and *Desired Goal* ratings for some of the components.

Less Healthy
Low Control/Willingness

Extremely Healthy
High Control/Willingness

| Incite & Accelerate | Slow Progression | Mitigate & Arrest | Prevent & Reverse |

10%   20   30   40   50%   60   70   80   90   100%

Overall Lifestyle Wellness Self-Evaluation. The decisions you make every day add up to impact your health and wellness in the long term. How do you want to live into the future – potentially disease free or taking a chance with your genetics - managing chronic diseases with medications, doctor's visits, and procedures. Being willing to do enough to move and sustain your Future Lifestyle Wellness Practices into the green range may increase your probability of adding years to your life and life to your years.

a) My Overall Lifestyle Wellness Current Baseline:	b) My Overall Lifestyle Wellness Desired Goal:	c) My Overall Willingness to Invest to Achieve My Lifestyle Wellness Desired Goal:	d) My Overall Lifestyle Wellness Future Target:
39	81	90	77

Example: Overall Lifestyle Wellness average ratings.

3. Complete the Courage & Confidence Check.

Your courage and confidence may impact your willingness to invest in your wellness journey. You're open to keeping a growth mindset, you've identified your baseline for each component, and you've chosen your goal, yet you still may feel hesitant or unsure about your ability to pull it off. It's normal that you may still feel a bit unwilling to make changes.

Willingness can be enhanced by feeling prepared. You may feel this way because you are not yet fully prepared. However, as you complete additional sections of your *Lifestyle Wellness Strategic Plan*, your path to the health and wellness you desire will become more tangible and doable in your mind, and you will feel more prepared to take the next steps.

a. I must warn you that the level of planning needed to achieve your desired health and wellness will most likely be at a level you've never done before. You may be used to this in your work world, but not as it relates to your health and wellness.

Using a scale of 1-10 (with 10 being Extremely Courageous and 1 being Not Very Courageous At All), how **courageous** do you feel about moving further into the process to plan your wellness at a high level of detail to achieve the health and wellness you desire?

My **courage** level is:

1   2   3   4   5   6   7   8   9   10

What influenced my rating choice?

_____

_____

If my rating is less than 7, I will take the following actions to increase my **courage** level to get ready to go deep into my planning to achieve the health and wellness I desire:

_____

_____

b. How **confident** do you feel that you can do it? Many people think planning is stifling and not their thing. They may shut down when it comes to planning, avoid it altogether, and simply wing it. Unfortunately, failing to plan equals planning to fail. This may be why you've struggled with your health and wellness. It helps to think of your plan as a way to organize your thinking and wrap your hands and heart around achieving the health and wellness you envision; you are still in control of the level of detail you want to put in each section.

Using a scale of 1-10 (with 10 being Extremely Confident and 1 being Not Very Confident At All), how **confident** do you feel about staying engaged with your wellness planning to complete the remaining sections of your plan?

My **confidence** level is:

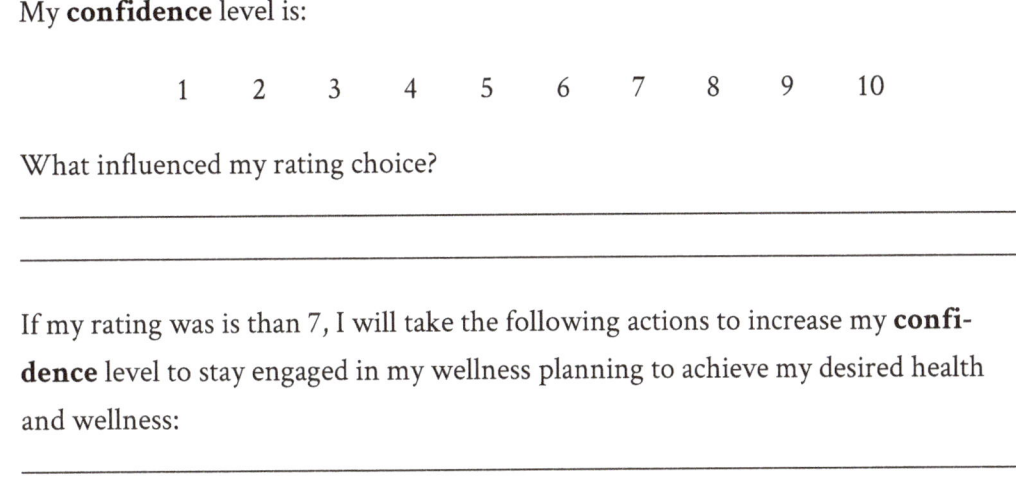

What influenced my rating choice?

_____

_____

If my rating was is than 7, I will take the following actions to increase my **confidence** level to stay engaged in my wellness planning to achieve my desired health and wellness:

_____

_____

4. **How confident are you in your self-ratings?** Sometimes it's difficult to be objective using a self-rating scale. You may be too harsh or not harsh enough.

Complete my detailed online assessment to evaluate your Current and Future Reality, which includes a body systems analysis with chronic disease progression risk and lifestyle wellness component impacts.

NOTE: Access the link to the assessment in the Week 5 section of the book resource website.

NOTES & QUESTIONS TO BE ANSWERED

WEEK 6

ORGANIZE YOUR LIFESTYLE OF WELLNESS INVESTING

How everyday people build extraordinary health and wellness.

"Good health is not something we can buy. However, it can be an extremely valuable savings account."

-ANNE WILSON SCHAEF, AUTHOR AND PSYCHIATRIST

It's time to begin elevating your health to that of your wealth. One without the other is not a great place to be. **Don't wait until you lose your health before you decide to value it!** Unfortunately, most people do.

Does your health & wellness sometimes feel like a cluttered, disorganized closet? You've "tried on" many solutions and programs over the years; some fit well and brought you joy, others not so much. Some may no longer fit; you keep adding to your closet, and you're not sure what you have in there anymore. You keep wearing the same things and expecting different results, hoping to fit back into some of your old things.

Your *Lifestyle Wellness Strategic Plan* is your vision of your redesigned and reorganized wellness closet, what you keep, what you eliminate, what new possibilities you add, and how you feel every morning when trying things on.

In **Week 6**, you get to begin **organizing your wellness closet to support your authentic level of wellness joy**, regardless of what is going on in your life. You redesign your wellness so you **never revert to clutter again**. You get to clear the clutter and decide how to do *authentic you*.

| 12 |

Your Lifestyle Wellness Strategic Plan

Organize and reorganize your authentic wellness journey of a lifetime.

It's time for your new beginning. **It's time for a release of new energy in a new direction toward achieving your best self.**

Your *Lifestyle Wellness Strategic Plan* is here to support your authentic journey. Organizing your journey in your *Lifestyle Wellness Strategic Plan* makes your *Wellness Vision* tangible.

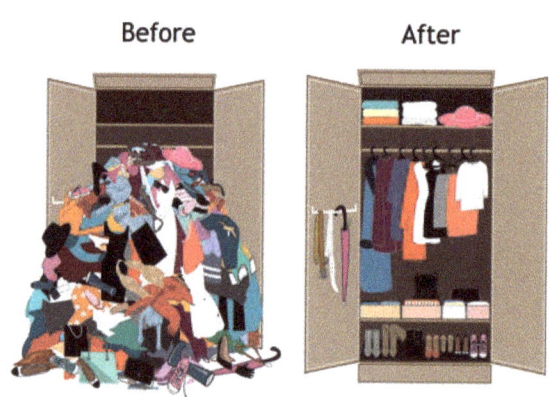

Before   After

Organize your wellness journey to feel like the closet on the right.

I like to use a closet metaphor to describe what this feels like. You reorganize your wellness closet to support your authentic level of wellness joy, regardless of what is going on in your life. Your authentic *Lifestyle Wellness Strategic Plan* provides that organization and includes accessories and resilience and contingency tactics to prevent your wellness closet from relapsing into disarray.

Documenting your plan and communicating your intentions to yourself and others increases your chances of achieving the wellness you desire by 80 percent. **Document and socialize your plan to make it real!**

Strategic Wellness Activities

In this chapter's strategic wellness activity, you complete the *first four sections* of your *Lifestyle Wellness Strategic Plan* using your inputs from previous chapters' activities. You get to enter the key inputs you've developed thus far. Use the following steps so you can compile a strong wellness foundation to build upon for the remaining sections of your plan.

1. Download the *Lifestyle Wellness Strategic Plan* template.

You will use this template to enter the key inputs you've developed thus far as well as enter your planning work for the remaining chapters.

> NOTE: Download the PDF fillable *Lifestyle Wellness Strategic Plan* template in the Week 6 section on the book resource website.

2. Complete Section 1.0: My Wellness Mission, Vision, & Aspirations.

This section presents your overall, lasting formulation of why you want to embark on your wellness journey and what you envision you will become. It paints a picture of where you want your health and wellness to be in the future. By making your wellness mission, vision, and aspirations concrete, you are taking a significant first step toward creating a plan that can lead you to success.

The inputs for this section come from the following strategic wellness activities in:

- Chapter 3: Why Now? Uncovering Your True Wellness Why

- Chapter 8: Visualizing Your Future Direction

- Chapter 9: The Reality of the Future You

Enter the following items into the template fields (see following example):

a. *Wellness Why* for your Mission statement.
b. The name you chose for your Road to Change is your *Wellness Journey Aspiration*.
c. *Wellness Vision* for your Vision statement.

1.0 My Wellness Mission, Vision, & Aspirations

My Wellness Mission (Wellness Why):
To be fit, strong, and in control, living a long, vibrant, disease-free life so I can be here to care for my parents and my family and pay it forward by becoming a wellness role model and support for others.

My Wellness Journey Aspiration: Energizing Lifestyle Lane

My Wellness Vision:
I review my Wellness Vision often to help me stay committed to becoming a healthy role model for my family, friends, and clients. I integrate wellness activities throughout my entire day, so I am not losing time away from my family and work. I include my family when possible, so we have fun together and stay engaged. I make continuous changes to my work and home environments to make healthy choices easy and effortless. I use my wellness strategic plan to keep me confident that the evidence-based choices I make every day have the potential to reverse and prevent chronic diseases of lifestyle and support longevity. I make time for self-care every day to manage my stress and wake up energetic, motivated, and ready to take on whatever the day brings.

Example: Section 1.0 from my Lifestyle Wellness Strategic Plan

3. Complete Section 2.0: My Wellness Authenticity.

This section highlights the core strengths and values that will guide your day-to-day and long-range decision-making about your health choices. When your decisions align with your strengths and values, your actions feel authentic, enjoyable, and effortless. Solidify your strengths in your mind and be creative when aligning all wellness activities with your strengths.

The inputs for this section come from the strategic wellness activity in:

- Chapter 4: You Have What It Takes - Your Wellness Authenticity

Enter the following items into the template fields (see following example):

a. Your strengths in Column 1.
b. In Column 2, how you will leverage each strength to achieve the wellness you desire.

2.0 My Wellness Authenticity

My Top Strengths & Values	I Will Leverage This Strength/Value to Support My Strategic Wellness Journey by:
Ideation (Creativity)	Identifying creative ways and endless possiblities to integrate activity into my current day without adding extra time to my already busy schedule.
Maximizer	Not doing anything half way, always committing to having the best experience possible without letting external events and other people affect my forward progress.

Example: Section 2.0 from my Lifestyle Wellness Strategic Plan

4. Complete Section 3.0: My Wellness Presence.

This section contains your RICE Analysis. These four components support your ability to stay focused and motivated along your health and wellness journey. Your goal is to increase all components concurrently to achieve balance.

You should continuously monitor your RICE components so you can feel when any of the components are falling out of balance. An imbalance can happen at any time throughout your lifetime wellness journey.

The inputs for this section come from the strategic wellness activity in:

■ Chapter 5: Finding & Strengthening Your Wellness Presence - Activity #1

Transcribe the following items into the template fields (see following example):

a. Check the box to indicate your rating for each RICE component (Activity #1, Column a.).
b. In the space next to each component, what new thoughts will keep each rating balanced and elevated (Activity #1, Column d.).
c. Add additional tactics as needed to support balanced and elevated RICE levels.

When you begin designing the tactics to achieve your wellness goals and targets, your design should include distractions and ways to enhance your readiness, importance, confidence, and enthusiasm integrated with your tactics.

3.0 My Wellness Presence - RICE Analysis

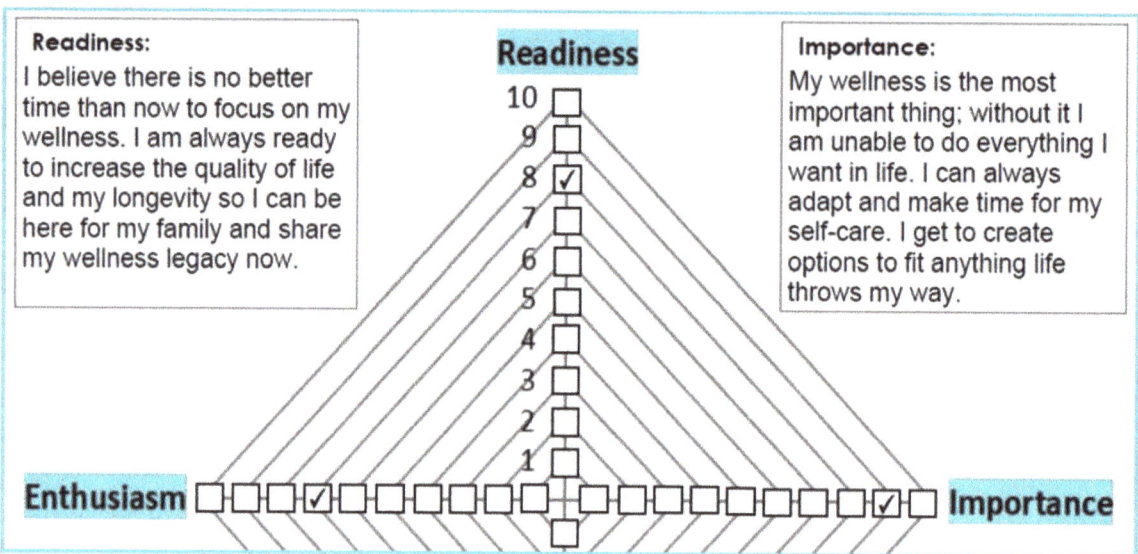

Readiness:
I believe there is no better time than now to focus on my wellness. I am always ready to increase the quality of life and my longevity so I can be here for my family and share my wellness legacy now.

Importance:
My wellness is the most important thing; without it I am unable to do everything I want in life. I can always adapt and make time for my self-care. I get to create options to fit anything life throws my way.

Example: Section 3.0 from my Lifestyle Wellness Strategic Plan

5. Complete Section 4.0: My Lifestyle Wellness Investment Goals & Targets.

This section provides awareness and insight – an internal perspective – into how your lifestyle choices impact your body systems' health and wellness; it's not just about what you see externally.

The inputs for this section come from the strategic wellness activity in:

■ Chapter 10: Your Current Reality
■ Chapter 11: How Much Will You Invest?

Your candid self-ratings present a snapshot that is the most valuable and revealing for you. This section represents your long-range wellness goals and targets and shows what you get to concentrate on to align your tactics with your *Wellness Why* and bring your *Wellness Vision* to life.

Through the lifestyle choices you decide you are willing to make, you have the potential to accelerate, slow, stop, prevent, and potentially reverse chronic diseases from setting in. In the evaluation, you decided how far you were willing to go, reflected in your *Future Targets*. Being willing to do enough to move and sustain your wellness practices into the green range increases your probability of adding years to your life and life to your years.

Enter the following items into the template fields (see following examples):

a. Transcribe your *Current Baseline* rating and *Future Target* rating from your worksheet into the associated columns for each Lifestyle Wellness component and enter your *Overall Lifestyle Wellness.*

b. Review your *Future Target* ratings - do they align with your *Wellness Vision?* Remember, these are the long-term targets you want to achieve. It may take a year or more to accomplish some of them. Be sure they align with your vision. Are you okay with potentially slowing the progression of chronic diseases of lifestyle, or would you prefer to do more to potentially stop or reverse them in 5 years? Are your targets too optimistic for you? Adjust your *Future Targets* as necessary to ensure they feel authentic to you. In the next chapter, you may feel more comfortable setting *Interim Goals* to take smaller steps toward achieving your *Future Targets.*

	Incite & Accelerate		Slow Progression		Mitigate & Arrest		Prevent & Reverse	
	10%	20	30	40	50%	60	70	80	90	100%
NUTRITION		20				56				

Example: Section 4.0 Current Baseline & Future Target values

	Incite & Accelerate		Slow Progression		Mitigate & Arrest		Prevent & Reverse	
	10%	20	30	40	50%	60	70	80	90	100%
Overall Lifestyle Wellness			39				77			

Example: Section 4.0 Overall Lifestyle Wellness Current Baseline & Future Target

6. Complete the Courage & Confidence Check.

Your **courage** and **confidence** affect where you set your *Future Targets* for each Lifestyle Wellness component. Taking a long-term, strategic, internal perspective of your health and wellness is not always easy.

a. **It's not always easy to admit that your actions are inciting and accelerating chronic diseases and unhealthy aging in your body.** It may be easier to avoid thinking about what you can't see happening inside your body, or it may seem like an impact that is years away. But, as you learned at the start of your journey, it is not normal to grow old with chronic diseases – chronic diseases develop from taking small, consistent, unhealthy actions over time.

Using a scale of 1-10 (with 10 being Extremely Courageous and 1 being Not Very Courageous At All), how **courageous** do you feel about taking an internal perspective and admitting that your life choices may be negatively impacting your health and wellness ?

My **courage** level is:

1   2   3   4   5   6   7   8   9   10

What influenced my rating choice?

_____

_____

If my rating is less than 7, I will take the following actions to increase my **courage** level to take an internal perspective and admit to the consequences of my actions:

_____

_____

b. How **confident** do you feel that you can achieve the *Future Targets* you've chosen? Now that you see the internal impact of your actions, it may be easier to commit to making enough changes to achieve your desired health and wellness.

Using a scale of 1-10 (with 10 being Extremely Confident and 1 being Not Very Confident At All), how **confident** do you feel that you can achieve the *Future Targets* you've chosen?

My **confidence** level is:

1   2   3   4   5   6   7   8   9   10

What influenced my rating choice?

_____

_____

If my rating is less than 7, I will take the following actions to increase my **confidence** level to achieve the Future Targets I've chosen:

_____

_____

NOTES & QUESTIONS TO BE ANSWERED

| 13 |

The Lifestyle of Wellness Investing

Stack the deck in favor of you having a long healthspan and lifespan.

Lifestyle Wellness Investing **shifts your focus to the long-life game by you taking charge of your health and wellness destiny in the present.** It gives you an internal perspective of your health and wellness by examining body systems (e.g., cardiovascular, digestive, urinary, immune, etc.), metabolic health, and longevity.

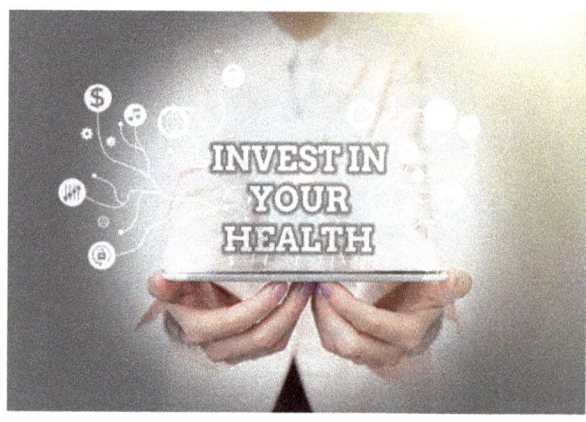

The healthy person you want to be won't happen by accident. Who do you want to be ten years from now, and what are the chances it is just going to happen? The same is true with your wealth. A life wealthy in resources, relationships, and purpose does not happen on its own.

You've most likely seen references to the greatest wealth is health, but what does that actually mean? It means treating **your health and wellness as an investment strategy for retirement and beyond** and benefiting from it now without interest and penalties for early distribution" (and no Form 1099-R to file).

Strategic Wellness Activities

In this chapter's strategic wellness activities, you will continue to refine your goals and targets to make them feel authentic and doable. You may decide you feel more comfortable with small-increment, 6-month *Interim Goals*.

I suggest setting an *Interim Goal* **if the gap between your** *Current Baseline* **and** *Future Target* **is greater than 20 percent**; however, if you are *Willing to Invest* and go all in, there is no need to set an *Interim Goal*, but this is a strategy that potentially increases your risk for burn out and relapse.

NOTE: Use your *Lifestyle Wellness Strategic Plan* you started in the previous chapter. The plan template is located in the Week 6 section on the book resource website.

1. Set 6-month *Interim Goals* **for each lifestyle wellness component.**

Return to *Section 4.0 in your Lifestyle Wellness Strategic Plan.*

a. **For each lifestyle wellness component, examine the gap between your** *Current Baseline* **and** *Future Target.* The percentage level on the continuum means that you choose to align your behaviors with that percentage level of the standard.

b. **Next, enter your** *Interim Goal* **for components with more significant gaps and for components you would like to progress slower** (see the following example). You may decide to readjust your goals and targets again when you begin detailed planning in Part 3. Again, nothing is set in stone; iteration and experimentation are the keys to achieving authenticity.

- **What feels realistic to you, given where you are in your life and what you have going on at home and work?** You are in charge! Don't take on more than you can handle right now. Sometimes a smaller, more realistic, and achievable goal will help you get started on a positive note.

- If you are ready to go all in and have a smaller gap to close between your *Current Baseline* and *Future Target,* shoot for your *Future Target* and enter the same value as your 6-month *Interim Goal.* Choose an *Interim Goal* whenever you would prefer to take more time to transition.

- Achieving and sustaining some of your long-range *Future Targets* may take time and additional 6-month *Interim Goal* iterations to transition effectively and achieve your targets fully. That's why you should think of your *Lifestyle Wellness Strategic Plan* as a living, breathing document that you review periodically and update as you achieve your *Interim Goals* and *Future Targets* and when your life situation changes. It may work best for you to focus on some components fully and make smaller changes in other areas. All components are interrelated. Research supports that improving your nutrition, movement, and sleep will have an indirect, positive effect on your mood and stress resistance.

	Incite & Accelerate			Slow Progression		Mitigate & Arrest		Prevent & Reverse	

	10%	20	30	40	50%	60	70	80	90	100%
NUTRITION		20		40		56				

Example: Section 4.0 Creating an Interim Goal

2. Complete the Courage and Confidence Check.

Your **courage** and **confidence** affect where you set your 6-month *Interim Goals* and *Future Targets* for each Lifestyle Wellness component based on your awareness of the *Evidence-Based Quality Standards* you want to work toward.

a. It's not always easy to predict the future – life has a way of interrupting even the best-laid plans.

Using a scale of 1-10 (with 10 being Extremely Courageous and 1 being Not Very Courageous At All), how **courageous** do you feel about taking the next steps toward achieving your 6-month goals for each component?

My **courage** level is:

1   2   3   4   5   6   7   8   9   10

What influenced my rating choice?

_____

_____

If my rating is less than 7, I will take the following actions to increase my **courage** level to take the next steps toward achieving my 6-month *Interim Goals:*

_____

_____

b. How **confident** do you feel that you can achieve the 6-month *Interim Goals* you've chosen? Having evidence-based goals and guidelines will improve your **confidence** that you are doing the right things in the right amount to achieve your expectations about your health and wellness goals. In addition, you now have the information to level-set your actions with your expectations.

Using a scale of 1-10 (with 10 being Extremely Confident and 1 being Not Very Confident At All), how **confident** do you feel that you can achieve the 6-month *Interim Goals* you've chosen?

My **confidence** level is:

1   2   3   4   5   6   7   8   9   10

What influenced my rating choice?

_____

_____

If my rating is less than 7, I will take the following actions to increase my **confidence** level to achieve the 6-month *Interim Goals* I've chosen:

_____

_____

NOTES & QUESTIONS TO BE ANSWERED

WEEK 7

YOUR LIFESTYLE WELLNESS INTERNAL FOUNDATION

Take great care of your body; it's the only one you have.

"No matter what the magazines at the supermarket checkout may say, we really could never make our skin healthy or our hair, our hearts, or brains, or eyes without simply eating to make ourselves healthy—a diet of wholesome foods in a sensible combination feeds all bits of us."

-DR. DAVID KATZ

Well-Leaders believe that lifestyle practices and health habits are the most important determinants of positive health. They take charge of their health and wellness destiny using evidence-based lifestyle medicine practices. They role-model lifestyle wellness themselves and pay it forward to others.

Your mind is your instrument for extraordinary health and wellness. You don't get what you want in life; you get who you are! You don't need a new day to start over; you only need a new mindset.

You should never take action from your present thought. Instead, you must take action from your future beliefs. Present thought creates the same old results. Future beliefs create endless possibilities. It's time to start living the vision of your future wellness.

In **Week 7**, you get to decide how you want to **take care of and nurture your body** with healthful nutrition, consistent movement, and quality sleep by **balancing the *evidence-based quality standards*** to fit your authentic life of wellness.

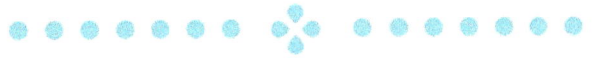

| 14 |

Your Lifestyle Wellness Roadmap – Eat, Move, Sleep (EMS)

Our bodies crave healthful, balanced nutrition, consistent movement, and adequate sleep to perform efficiently, heal, regenerate, and recharge.

Y ou are NOT at the mercy of your genetics! **You get to change your destiny**. How much are you willing to invest to increase the probability that your actions and habits are contributing to a long, disease-free lifespan by mindfully integrating lifestyle wellness into everything you do?

Are you ready to take the first steps toward living the new you?

Of all the lifestyle medicine components, Eat, Move, and Sleep (EMS) would be great priorities to start your planning. That's why I included the acronym EMS in the chapter title, to reflect their urgency and importance.

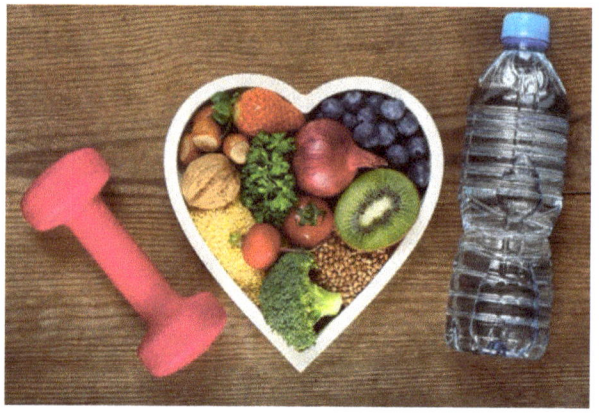
Balance your tactics for nutrition, movement, & sleep.

Strategic Wellness Activities

1. Complete the Nutrition, Movement, and Sleep Quality Planning worksheet.

The planning worksheet explains each *EBQS* in more detail and describes how to interpret and balance your *Interim Goal* percentages. Apply the formula(s) to guide the development of your daily, weekly, and monthly tactics and distractions that feel authentic to you.

2. Reconfirm your *Future Target* and 6-month *Interim Goal* percentages and select your tactics and distractions.

Your tactics and distractions are what you get to use to achieve your goals for wholesome **Nutrition**, consistent **Movement**, and improved **Sleep Quality**. Remember, your *Interim Goal* percentages represent the level of the *EBQS* you have chosen for each lifestyle wellness component that supports your *Wellness Vision.*

For example, if your *Interim Goal for* Nutrition is 60 percent, you choose tactics and distractions to reinforce achieving a 60 percent predominately whole food, plant-based nutritional plan over the next six months.

3. Update Section 5.0 in your *Lifestyle Wellness Strategic Plan.*

Transcribe your *Future Targets* and *Interim Goals* for Nutrition, Movement, and Sleep in this section (see the example below).

LIFESTYLE COMPONENT		MY TACTICS (daily, weekly, monthly)	MY STRENGTHS-BASED DISTRACTIONS
1	**Lifestyle Nutrition**		
Future Target:	56		
6-Month Interim Goal:	40		
EBQS: Optimize healthy, micronutrient-dense food choices using evidence-based dietary practices that include predominantly • Whole Plant Foods • Minimally processed • High in fiber • Low in added salt, sugar, and oil • Low in saturated fat			

Section 5.0 Wellness Investor Mindset Tactics & Distractions

4. Enter your tactics and distractions into your plan.

Document the initial tactics and distractions you will use to achieve your *Interim Goals* for wholesome Nutrition, consistent Movement, and improved quality Sleep.

> NOTE: See the Week 7 section on the book resource website for Lifestyle Medicine Guidelines, tips, and suggestions to help you develop your initial tactics and distractions.

5. Complete the Courage & Confidence Check.

How did you do with creating your tactics and distractions for these components? Do your tactics and distractions for these components reflect your **courage** to step out of your comfort zone and try new things? How will your distraction(s) keep you on track and motivated?

a. You've learned about evidence-based actions to support Nutrition, Movement, and Sleep, and what makes the tactics you've chosen feel new, innovative, and aligned with your strengths.

Using a scale of 1-10 (with 10 being Extremely Courageous and 1 being Not Very Courageous At All), how **courageous** are you feeling about implementing your tactics and distractions for these components and stepping out of your comfort zone?

My **courage** level is:

1   2   3   4   5   6   7   8   9   10

What influenced my rating choice?

_____

_____

If my rating is less than 7, I will take the following actions to increase my **courage** level to implement my tactics and distractions for Nutrition, Movement, & Sleep enough to step out of my comfort zone:

_____

_____

b. Aligning your tactics and distractions for the Nutrition, Movement, and Sleep components with your strengths will increase your **confidence** in your ability to step out of your comfort zone and sustain your lifelong journey. Staying aligned with your strengths and values ensures you do what you enjoy and keeps you motivated to sustain your health and wellness goals.

Using a scale of 1-10 (with 10 being Extremely Confident and 1 being Not Very Confident At All), how **confident** do you feel that you have aligned your tactics with your strengths and values to achieve and sustain the 6-month *Interim Goals* you've chosen?

My **confidence** level is:

1   2   3   4   5   6   7   8   9   10

What influenced my rating choice?

_____

_____

If my rating is less than 7, I will take the following actions to continue increasing my **confidence** level that my tactics are aligned with my strengths and values to achieve and sustain the 6-month _Interim Goals_ I've chosen:

_____

_____

Nutritional Quality Planning

Nutrition plays a substantial role in almost every aspect of one's life. Better overall health and body composition are attributable *to improvements in healthy, nutrient-dense food choices* and *evidence-based dietary practices.*

Evidence-Based Quality Standard: To optimize the percentage of **WEEKLY** intake of 3 main meals and 2 snacks per day that are **Whole Plant-Based Foods** with

- High micronutrient density
- Minimal processing
- Low added salt, oil, & sugar
- Low saturated fat
- And, avoid sugary beverages

Circle your current Nutrition Interim Goal %

FEWER WHOLE PLANT-BASED FOODS						MORE WHOLE PLANT-BASED-FOODS			
10%	20	30	40	50%	60	70	80	90	100%
Incite & Accelerate				Slow Progression		Mitigate & Arrest			Prevent & Reverse

EBQS Balancing Formula

Choose one of the options below or a combination that works for you.

Option 1: Percentage of Weekly Meals

Main meals per WEEK _____ x Interim Goal % _____ = # Whole food, plant-based meals per WEEK _____.

Snacks per WEEK _____ x Interim Goal % _____ = # Whole food, plant-based snacks per WEEK _____.

Beverages per WEEK _____ x Interim Goal % _____ = # Unsweetened beverages per WEEK _____.

Option 2: Meal Composition Percentage

Interim Goal % _____ = the composition percentage of main meals and snacks per WEEK that are whole food, plant based (e.g., 60% of food on the plate or snack is whole-food, plant-based).

For Beverages, use Option 1.

Nutrition Quality Tactics & Distractions

Enter your tactics and distractions to achieve your balanced Nutrition Quality *Interim Goal* percentage. Transcribe your tactics and distractions into your *Lifestyle Wellness Strategic Plan.* This is your starting point when implementing your plan.

Nutrition Quality Tactics	Nutrition Quality Distractions

Total Movement Quality Planning

Exercise is medicine. An overwhelming body of evidence supports that significant mental and physical health benefits are attributable to *regular weekly structured exercise, unstructured movement and less sitting*.

Evidence-Based Quality Standard: To increase regular **WEEKLY** movement to achieve total body fitness through

Structured Exercise Movement Minimum (SEMM) – WEEKLY percentage of achievement of 150-min of moderate-intensity cardiovascular activity, 75-min of vigorous intensity, or a combination of the two; plus, resistance training x 2, stretching x 3, and balance/agility training daily.

Daily Sitting – Percentage of waking hours spent sitting for meals, work, and lifestyle activities (television watching, gaming, events, sporting and household activities, etc.).

Circle your current SEMM Interim Goal %.

< 25% SEMM	50% SEMM	100% OR > SEMM

10%	20	30	40	50%	60	70	80	90	100%
Incite & Accelerate				Slow Progression		Mitigate & Arrest		Prevent & Reverse	

Circle your current Sitting/Non-Structured Movement Interim Goal %.

> 9 HRS/DAY	7-8 HRS/DAY	5-6 HRS/DAY	< 4 HRS/DAY

10%	20	30	40	50%	60	70	80	90	100%
Incite & Accelerate				Slow Progression		Mitigate & Arrest		Prevent & Reverse	

EBQS Balancing Formula

Scale your monthly and weekly total body fitness using the formulas below.

Structured Exercise Movement:

- **Cardiovascular: 150 min** x Interim Goal % = _____ minutes per WEEK of moderate intensity OR **75 min** x Interim Goal % = _____ minutes per WEEK of vigorous intensity (or combination)
- **Resistance/Weight Training**: **2-3 times per WEEK** x Interim Goal % = _____ times per WEEK of resistance training
- **Stretching**: **3 times per WEEK** x Interim Goal % = _____ times per WEEK of stretching
- **Agility Training**: **7 times per WEEK** x Interim Goal % = _____ times per WEEK of balance and agility training

Non-Structured/Sitting:

- Interim Goal % = _____ per DAY. Work toward sitting less than _____ HOURS per Day. Estimate your hours per day based on the location of your *Interim Goal* % on the chronic disease progression range.

Movement Quality Tactics & Distractions

Enter your tactics and distractions to achieve your balanced Movement Quality *Interim Goal* percentage. Transcribe your tactics and distractions into your *Lifestyle Wellness Strategic Plan.* This is your starting point when implementing your plan.

Structured Movement Quality Tactics	Structured Movement Quality Distractions

Sitting/Unstructured Movement Quality Tactics	Sitting/Unstructured Movement Quality Distractions

Sleep Quality Planning

Optimal sleep is a learned behavior. Improving sleep quality is attributable to *entraining your internal body clock* (circadian rhythm) by making evidence-based, proactive changes to your sleep routine and environment, light exposure and timing, food and beverage intake, and stress management.

Evidence-Based Quality Standard: To improve the WEEKLY quality of your sleep by entraining your internal body clock (circadian rhythm) to

Reduce Wake-Sleep Time: time it takes to fall asleep after your head hits the pillow.

Extend Sleep Periods: time spent in uninterrupted sleep without extended periods of wakefulness.

Maintain Efficient Sleep-Wake Time: achieving desired wake time without use of alarm.

Circle your current Wake-Sleep Time Interim Goal %.

> 3 HOURS	2 HOURS	1 HOUR	30 MINUTES	< 15 MINUTES

10%	20	30	40	50%	60	70	80	90	100%
Incite & Accelerate				Slow Progression		Mitigate & Arrest		Prevent & Reverse	

Circle your current Sleep Period Interim Goal %.

> 3 HOURS	4 HOURS	5 HOURS	6 HOURS	> 7 HOURS

10%	20	30	40	50%	60	70	80	90	100%
Incite & Accelerate				Slow Progression		Mitigate & Arrest		Prevent & Reverse	

Circle your current Sleep-Wake Time Interim Goal %.

> 2 HOURS	1 HOUR	30 MINUTES	< 15 MINUTES

10%	20	30	40	50%	60	70	80	90	100%
Incite & Accelerate				Slow Progression		Mitigate & Arrest		Prevent & Reverse	

EBQS Balancing Formula

Scale your weekly sleep quality using the formulas below. Estimate the hours or minutes for each attribute based on the location of the percentage on the chronic disease progression range.

Wake-Sleep Time:

- My Interim Goal % = _____. Work toward falling asleep within _____ HOURS or MINUTES of sleep initiation.

Sleep Periods:

- My Interim Goal % = _____. Work toward extending cumulative sleep periods to _____ HOURS per night.

Sleep-Wake Time:

- My Interim Goal % = _____. Work toward waking up within _____ HOURS or MINUTES of desired wake time without the use of an alarm and feeling alert/awake throughout the day.

Sleep Quality Tactics & Distractions

Enter your tactics and distractions to achieve your balanced Sleep Quality *Interim Goal* percentage. Transcribe your tactics and distractions into your *Lifestyle Wellness Strategic Plan*. This is your starting point when implementing your plan.

Wake-Sleep Quality Tactics	Wake-Sleep Quality Distractions

Sleep Periods Quality Tactics	Sleep Periods Quality Distractions

Sleep-Wake Quality Tactics	Sleep-Wake Quality Distractions

NOTES & QUESTIONS TO BE ANSWERED

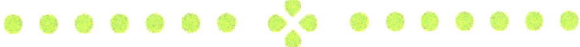

WEEK 8

YOUR LIFESTYLE WELLNESS EXTERNAL DEFENSE

Protect your body from external influences that can wreak havoc upon your immune system and increase chronic disease risk.

"Seventy percent of primary care provider visits are related to stress and lifestyle, and over 43 percent of adults suffer from adverse effects of unmanaged stress, which are linked to the development of chronic diseases."

-AMERICAN COLLEGE OF LIFESTYLE MEDICINE

External forces beyond your control have the potential to impact your long-term health and wellness. Unfortunately, the standard American lifestyle sets you up to be bombarded by these forces. When external forces become overwhelming, unhealthy coping mechanisms may automatically kick in. These include drinking alcohol, smoking, isolating oneself, losing purpose, or developing unhealthy relationships.

When experiencing stressful situations and encountering triggers, it is important to remember that external circumstances are not controlling your life unless you let them. You get to think about your present and your past in any way you want. This gets you out of the constant mind-drama and rumination about the past. The way you construct your thoughts gives the control back to you. Your beliefs and feelings create your actions and how you respond to external events. Thus, you always have a choice about how you adapt and respond to stress, create positivity and purpose in your life, experience situations, engage in relationships, and what substances and chemicals you expose your body to or choose to put into it.

In **Week 8**, you get to decide how to **use effective coping strategies**, **find purpose and meaning in your life**, and **minimize exposure to harmful substances** by balancing the evidence-based quality standards to fit your authentic life of wellness.

• • • • • • • • • ❖ • • • • • • • • •

Your Lifestyle Wellness Roadmap – De-Stress, Connect, Protect

The choice is always yours; however, nothing changes until you clean up your mind and 100% own what you are thinking and how you respond.

You continue to build on your wellness foundation by **protecting your body from external influences** that have the potential to wreak havoc upon your immune system and increase chronic disease risk for many body systems. The three culprits are managing stress, enhancing positivity & meaningful connections, and avoiding risky substances.

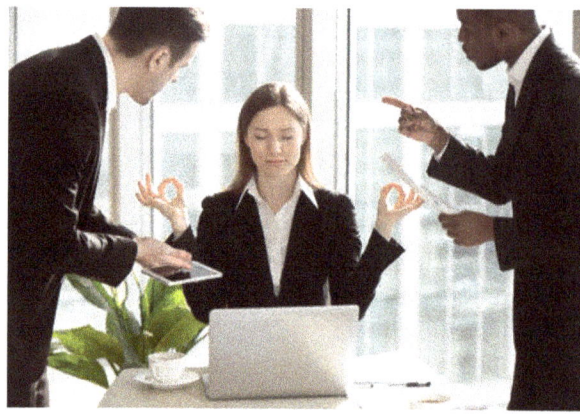

Tune out the noise and choose your future of possibilities.

You have the ability to **manage your response to your external environment** by creating tactics and distractions aligned with your new beliefs and thoughts about old habits and behavioral triggers.

Take responsibility and **stay out of the victim mentality** by not letting your external environment and the actions of others control you and not allowing events to trigger a negative response. Not succumbing to victim mode keeps you in charge of choosing a future of possibilities.

Strategic Wellness Activities

1. Review the Stress Management, Positivity & Social Connections, and Avoiding Risky Substances Quality Planning worksheet.

The planning worksheet explains each *EBQS* in more detail and describes how to interpret and balance your *Interim Goal* percentages. Apply the formula(s) to guide the development of your daily, weekly, and monthly tactics and distractions that feel authentic to you.

> NOTE: See the Week 8 section on the book resource website for the *Meaningful Connection Quality* assessment and the *Positive Possibilities Mindset* assessment to assist with setting *Interim Goals* and *Future Targets*.

2 Reconfirm your *Future Target* and 6-month *Interim Goal* percentages and select your tactics and distractions.

Your tactics and distractions are what you get to use to achieve your goals for effective stress management & elevated well-being, feeling connected with people and purpose, and protecting your body from damage caused by risky substances. Remember, your *Interim Goal* percentages represent the level of the EBQS you have chosen for each lifestyle wellness component that supports your *Wellness Vision*. For example, if your *Interim Goal* for Stress Management is 60 percent, you choose tactics and distractions to reinforce achieving 60 percent of your days each week in which you lower your stress levels using effective coping mechanisms over the next six months.

3. Update Section 5.0 in your *Lifestyle Wellness Strategic Plan*.

As you did in the previous chapter's activities, transcribe your *Future Targets* and *Interim Goals* for Stress Management, Positivity & Connections, and Avoiding Risky Substances into this section.

4. Enter your tactics and distractions into your plan.

Document the initial tactics and distractions you will use to achieve your balanced *Interim Goals* for Stress Management, Positivity & Connections, and Avoiding Risky Substances.

> NOTE: See the Week 8 section on the book resource website for Lifestyle Medicine Guidelines, tips, and suggestions to help you develop your initial tactics and distractions.

5. Complete the Courage & Confidence Check.

How did you do with creating your tactics and distractions for the Stress Management, Positivity & Connections, and Risky Substance Avoidance components? Do your tactics and distractions for these components reflect your **courage** to step out of your comfort zone and try new things? How do you feel your distraction(s) will help keep you on track and motivated?

a. You've learned about evidence-based actions to support stress reduction, connections and positivity, and avoidance of risky substances - what makes the tactics you've chosen feel NEW, innovative, and aligned with your strengths?

Using a scale of 1-10 (with 10 being Extremely Courageous and 1 being Not Very Courageous At All), how **courageous** are you feeling about implementing your tactics and distractions for these components and stepping out of your comfort zone?

My **courage** level is:

1   2   3   4   5   6   7   8   9   10

What influenced my rating choice?

_____

_____

If my rating is less than 7, I will take the following actions to increase my **courage** level to implement my tactics and distractions for Stress Reduction, Connections & Positivity, and Risky Substance Avoidance enough to step out of my comfort zone:

_____

_____

b. Aligning your tactics and distractions for the Stress Reduction, Connections & Positivity, and Risky Substance Avoidance components with your strengths and values will increase your **confidence** in your ability to achieve and sustain your lifelong journey. Staying aligned with your strengths and values will ensure you are doing the things you enjoy while keeping you motivated to sustain your health and wellness goals.

Using a scale of 1-10 (with 10 being Extremely Confident and 1 being Not Very Confident At All), how **confident** do you feel that you've aligned your tactics with your strengths enough to achieve and sustain the 6-month *Interim Goals* you've chosen?

My **confidence** level is:

1   2   3   4   5   6   7   8   9   10

What influenced your rating choice?

_____

_____

If my rating is less than 7, I will take the following actions to continue increasing my **confidence** level using tactics aligned with my strengths and values to achieve and sustain the 6-month *Interim Goals* I've chosen:

_____

_____

Stress Management Quality Planning

Stress is a constant in daily life. Improved mental well-being and better resiliency to manage stressful situations and fight the numerous symptoms and diseases associated with chronic stress are attributable to **developing healthy coping mechanisms**.

Evidence-Based Quality Standard: Optimize stress management and resilience by increasing:

> **Healthy Stress Adaptation** – Percentage over the past WEEK you felt in control of your responsibilities, your reactions to unexpected situations and your ability to use healthy coping strategies to handle personal and work issues that cause stress.

> **Balanced Mental Well-being** – Percentage over the past WEEK you felt free from anxiety, worry, depressed mood, and you experienced interest or pleasure in doing things.

Circle your current Stress Adaptation Interim Goal %

LOW ADAPTATION	MODERATE ADAPTATION	HIGH ADAPTATION

10%	20 ·	30	40	50%	60	70	80	90	100%
Incite & Accelerate				Slow Progression		Mitigate & Arrest		Prevent & Reverse	

Circle your current Mental Well-Being Interim Goal %

UNBALANCED WELL-BEING		BALANCED WELL-BEING

10%	20	30	40	50%	60	70	80	90	100%
Incite & Accelerate				Slow Progression		Mitigate & Arrest		Prevent & Reverse	

EBQS Balancing Formula

Healthy Stress Adaptation

- Interim Goal % _____ per WEEK you experience low stress, feel in control, and use healthy coping strategies. Use the **Perceived Stress Scale** on the book resource website to evaluate your weekly stress adaptation.

Balanced Mental Well-being

- Interim Goal % _____ per WEEK you feel balanced well-being, free from anxiety, worry, and/or depression. Use the **PHQ-4 Evaluation** on the book resource website to evaluate your weekly well-being.

Stress Management Quality Tactics & Distractions

Enter your tactics and distractions to achieve your Stress Management Quality *Interim Goal* percentage. Transcribe your tactics and distractions into your *Lifestyle Wellness Strategic Plan*. This is your starting point when implementing your plan.

Stress Adaptation Quality Tactics	Stress Adaptation Quality Distractions

Mental Well-Being Quality Tactics	Mental Well-Being Quality Distractions

Positivity & Social Connections Quality Planning

People need connections and a sense of belonging. An ongoing positive loop of social, emotional, and physical well-being is attributable to *engaging in and maintaining positive, balanced, healthy connections* personally and professionally. **Maintaining a positive possibilities mindset keeps you believing forward**, experiencing gratitude in the moment, and staying in an energy that attracts success.

Evidence-Based Quality Standard: Optimize positivity and social connections quality through:

Balancing Meaningful Connections - Connections percentage from the past WEEK in which you experienced balance with those people, places, things, ideas, information, and activities that provide positive feelings of connection.

Exhibiting a Positive Possibilties Mindset - Positive possibilties percentage from the past WEEK in which you experienced strong beliefs in your ability to manage your future success and reprogram your thoughts consistent with mindset transformation.

Circle your current Connections Interim Goal %

UNBALANCED CONNECTIONS							BALANCED CONNECTIONS		
10%	20	30	40	50%	60	70	80	90	100%
Incite & Accelerate				Slow Progression		Mitigate & Arrest		Prevent & Reverse	

Circle your current Positive Possiblities Mindset Interim Goal %

LOW POSITIVE POSSIBILITIES MINDSET						HIGH POSITIVE POSSIBILTIES MINDSET		
10%	20	30	40	50%	60	70	80	90	100%
Incite & Accelerate				Slow Progression		Mitigate & Arrest		Prevent & Reverse	

EBQS Balancing Formula

Balanced Meaningful Connections

- Interim Goal % = _____ per WEEK in which you experience balanced meaningful connections. Use the **Meaningful Connections Evaluation** on the book resource website to evaluate your weekly balance.

Positive Possibilties Mindset

- Interim Goal % = _____ per WEEK in which you exhibit a balanced positive possibilities mindset. Use the **Positive Possibilities Mindset Evaluation** on the book resource website to evaluate your weekly possibilities mindset.

Positivity & Connections Quality Tactics & Distractions

Enter your tactics and distractions to achieve your Positivity & Connections Quality *Interim Goal* percentage. Transcribe your tactics and distractions into your *Lifestyle Wellness Strategic Plan*. This is your starting point when implementing your plan.

Positivity & Social Connections Quality Tactics	Positivity & Social Connections Quality Tactics

Positive Possibilities Mindset Quality Tactics	Positive Possibilities Mindset Quality Distractions

Risky Substance Avoidance Quality Planning

People use and are prone to overusing a wide variety of substances, potentially damaging to most body systems. Improved physical, mental, and social health and enhanced productivity and performance are attributable to developing an effective substance management strategy.

Evidence-Based Quality Standard: Optimize your substance management strategy by

Avoiding Alcohol Use: Based on the **NIH's Alcohol Use Low-Risk Drinking Guidelines:** for men - have no more than 2 drinks per day and no more than 14 per week; for women - have no more than 1 drink per day and no more than 7 drinks per week. *Meeting this standard aligns with 30% on the continuum.*

Eliminating Tobacco & Other Risky Substances – complete avoidance of tobacco and all risky substances.

Circle your current Alcohol Avoidance Interim Goal %

HIGH RISK/BINGE	* LOW RISK		RARE USE	FULL AVOIDANCE	

10%	20	30	40	50%	60	70	80	90	100%
Incite & Accelerate				Slow Progression		Mitigate & Arrest			Prevent & Reverse

EBQS Balancing Formula

Alcohol Avoidance

- Interim Goal % = _____ per WEEK.
- *Minimum Interim Goal should be 30%. Work toward achieving at least 30%; however, research supports that total alcohol avoidance is better for health.
- **For each 10% increase in Interim Goal %, reduce daily and weekly consumption using the following scaling**
  - **30-40% = Women:** 1 drink per day and no more than 5 drinks per week; **Men:** 2 drinks per day and no more than 10 drinks per week.
  - **41-50% = Women:** 1 drink per day and no more than 3 drinks per week; **Men:** 2 drinks per day and no more than 5 drinks per week.
  - **51-60 = Women:** 1 drink per day and no more than 2 drinks per week; **Men:** 2 drinks per day and no more than 4 drinks per week.
  - **61-80% = Rare Use**
  - **81-100% = Total Avoidance**

Eliminating Tobacco & Other Risky Substances

- **Recommend Total Avoidance** - work with your healthcare provider, counselor, or organization to develop your quit plan.

Risky Substance Avoidance Tactics & Distractions

Enter your tactics and distractions to achieve your Risky Substance Avoidance Quality *Interim Goal* percentage. Transcribe your tactics and distractions into your *Lifestyle Wellness Strategic Plan*. This is your starting point when implementing your plan.

Alcohol Avoidance Quality Tactics	Alcohol Avoidance Quality Distractions

Risky Substance Avoidance Quality Tactics	Risky Substance Avoidance Quality Distractions

NOTES & QUESTIONS TO BE ANSWERED

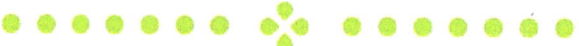

WEEK 9

YOUR LIFESTYLE WELLNESS SUPPORTIVE ENVIRONMENTS

To lead a life that includes extraordinary health and wellness, embrace Wellness Nonconformity in an unhealthy conforming world. You must have the courage and confidence to go against the grain.

"If you want to lead an extraordinary life, find out what the ordinary do—and don't do it."

-TOMMY NEWBERRY

What does it look like when you go against the grain? **It's about believing in your *Wellness Vision* and taking inspired actions that align with your vision.** By overcoming short-term, instant gratification, mainstream thinking, and external "should" pressures, you get to defend your *Wellness Nonconformity*.

Making supportive changes in your home and work environments softens the mainstream and external pressures. However, setting up your environments to support extraordinary health and wellness often means going against the grain by putting on your Wellness-Nonconformist shoes.

When you do this, you don't have to rely on willpower and brute force. You get to take the easy way out by setting up your life in a way that **makes the healthy options your default**, go-to options that align with living your *Wellness Vision*.

In **Week 9**, you get to call upon your **creativity and innovation to design your home and work environments** to support your lifestyle wellness journey and make it easy to live your best self for life.

| 16 |

Your Lifestyle Wellness Roadmap – Support & Thrive

Living well and leading well by design creates the conditions in your brain to believe, reframe, and take charge of your health and wellness your way!

It is essential to optimize your home and work environments and structure your days to minimize obstacles so you can make the changes you desire to support your *Wellness Vision* and achieve your best possible self.

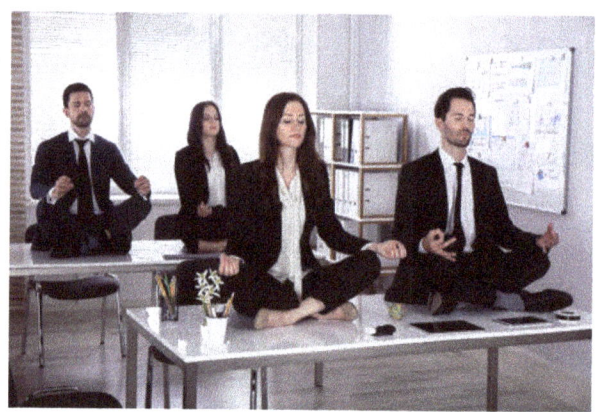

Let's face it, external things, events, and people are out of your control. Remember, however, nothing has to change in your external world for you to achieve the health and wellness you envision.

By creating supportive environments, essentially, you are deciding ahead of time who you are and how you roll every day. You show up how you want to show up. Things will throw you off, but you know what to go back to be-

Be the nonconformist well-leader of your team.

cause you believe in your *Wellness Vision* and get to make healthy choices your default option.

Strategic Wellness Activities

The strategic wellness activities in this chapter focus on how to optimize your home and work environments and structure your days to minimize obstacles so you can make the changes you desire to support your *Wellness Vision* and achieve your best possible self.

1. Review the Supportive Environments Planning worksheet.

The planning worksheet explains each *EBQS* in more detail and describes how to interpret and balance your *Interim Goal* percentages. Apply the formula(s) to guide the development of your daily, weekly, and monthly tactics and distractions that feel authentic to you.

2. Reconfirm your *Future Target* and 6-month *Interim Goal* percentages and select your tactics and distractions.

Your tactics and distractions are what you get to use to achieve your balanced *Interim Goals* for supportive environments. Remember, your *Interim Goal* percentages represent the level of the EBQS you have chosen for each lifestyle wellness component that supports your *Wellness Vision.*

> For example, if your *Interim Goal* for Supportive Home Environment is 60 percent, you choose tactics and distractions to reinforce achieving 60 percent of your days each week in which you feel your wellness is supported at home.

3. Complete Section 5.1: My Lifestyle Wellness By Design in your *Lifestyle Wellness Strategic Plan.*

Transcribe your *Future Targets* and *Interim Goals* for Supportive Home & Work Environments in this section.

4. Enter your tactics and distractions into your plan.

Document the initial tactics and distractions you will use to achieve your *Interim Goals* for supportive home and work environments.

> NOTE: See the Week 9 section on the book resource website for Lifestyle Wellness by Design Suggestions to help you develop your initial tactics and distractions.

5. Conduct a final review of Sections 5.0 and 5.1 in your plan.

These sections should be complete. For all eight lifestyle wellness components, confirm that you have entered all your *Interim Goals*, *Future Targets*, and the tactics and distractions you are willing to invest in over the next six months. Make adjustments to ensure your tactics and distractions feel authentic to you.

6. Complete the Courage & Confidence Check.

How did you do with creating your tactics and distractions for the Supportive Home & Work Environment components? Do your tactics and distractions for these components reflect your

courage to step out of your comfort zone and try new things? How do you feel your distraction(s) will help keep you on track and motivated?

a. You've learned about evidence-based actions to create supportive home and work environments - what makes the tactics you've chosen feel NEW, innovative, and aligned with your strengths?

Using a scale of 1-10 (with 10 being Extremely Courageous and 1 being Not Very Courageous At All), how **courageous** are you feeling about implementing your tactics and distractions for these components and stepping out of your comfort zone?

My **courage** level is:

1   2   3   4   5   6   7   8   9   10

What influenced my rating choice?

_____

_____

If my rating is less than 7, I will take the following actions to increase my **courage** level to implement my tactics and distractions for Supportive Home & Work Environments enough to step out of my comfort zone:

_____

_____

b. Aligning your tactics and distractions for the Supportive Home & Work Environment components with your strengths will increase your **confidence** in your ability to achieve and sustain your lifelong journey. Staying aligned with your strengths and values will ensure you are doing the things you enjoy while keeping you motivated to sustain your health and wellness goals.

Using a scale of 1-10 (with 10 being Extremely Confident and 1 being Not Very Confident At All), how **confident** do you feel that you've aligned your tactics with your strengths and values enough to achieve and sustain the 6-month *Interim Goals* you've chosen?

My **confidence** level is:

1   2   3   4   5   6   7   8   9   10

What influenced my rating choice?

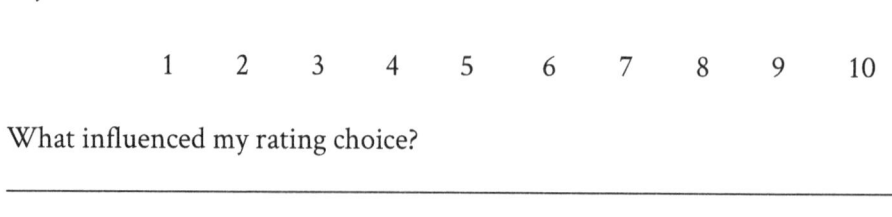

If my rating is less than 7, I will take the following actions to continue increasing my **confidence** level using tactics aligned with my strengths and values to achieve and sustain the 6-month *Interim Goals* I've chosen:

_____

_____

Supportive Environments Quality Planning

Your home and work environments must support your health and wellness. Health and wellness motivation, resilience, and sustainment are attributable to *designing work and home environments that limit the use of willpower and make healthy choices the default*.

Evidence-Based Quality Standard: Optimize and *design your life to elevate and support wellness* by making *healthy choices the default* and *prioritizing self-care* through

Supportive Home Life – Percentage of Days in the past WEEK you felt supported at home and did not put your engagement in healthy behaviors and self-care you had desired and planned on hold to care for others.

Supportive Work Life – Percentage of Days in the past WEEK you felt supported at work and you were able to integrate and engage in the wellness behaviors and self-care you had desired and planned.

Circle your current Supportive Home Environment Interim Goal %.

UNSUPPORTIVE HOME LIFE									SUPPORTIVE HOME LIFE
10%	20	30	40	50%	60	70	80	90	100%
Incite & Accelerate				Slow Progression		Mitigate & Arrest		Prevent & Reverse	

Circle your current Supportive Work Environment Interim Goal %.

UNSUPPORTIVE WORK LIFE									SUPPORTIVE WORK LIFE
10%	20	30	40	50%	60	70	80	90	100%
Incite & Accelerate				Slow Progression		Mitigate & Arrest		Prevent & Reverse	

EBQS Balancing Formula

Supportive Home Life

- Interim Goal % _____ x 7 DAYS = _____ Days/WEEK you feel supported at home to engage in self-care and wellness activities.

Supportive Work Life

- Interim Goal % _____ x 7 DAYS = _____ Days/WEEK you feel supported at work to engage in self-care and wellness activities.

Supportive Environments Tactics & Distractions

Enter your tactics and distractions to achieve your Supportive Environments Quality *Interim Goal* percentage. Transcribe your tactics and distractions into your *Lifestyle Wellness Strategic Plan*. This is your starting point when implementing your plan.

Supportive Home Environment Quality Tactics	Supportive Home Environment Quality Distractions

Supportive Work Environment Quality Tactics	Supportive Work Environment Quality Distractions

NOTES & QUESTIONS TO BE ANSWERED

WEEK 10

OPTIMIZE YOUR WELLNESS INVESTMENT

Invest in your wellness like your life depends on it because it does!

"Wise is wonderful, but probably sets the bar too high. We could be both healthy and wealthy - or at least exercise comparable control over both - if we were just comparably sensible about both health and wealth. Let's give it a try, shall we?"

-DR. DAVID KATZ

Think of your final plan as the **starting point for your wellness journey**. As with any plan, even in business, you want to know if your plan is consistently working for you after you've implemented it. Are you achieving the value and return on your wellness investments? Are you making progress toward achieving your lifestyle wellness *Future Targets*?

Health is a priceless wealth. I can't say it enough because I get to experience it now and will consistently defend my "Whealth."

How will you know if you are optimizing your investment in your lifelong health and wellness? You do this by treating your lifestyle wellness journey more like you do your wealth, investing in your *Wellness Vision* for the long term, and valuing your health while you are gaining it, not just focusing on it after you lose it.

In **Week 10**, you get to decide how to **monitor and manage your wellness investments.** Then, you optimize the return on your investments to keep you moving toward your *Wellness Vision* and know when to make adjustments to **grow and adapt** to what life throws your way.

| 17 |

Your Lifestyle Wellness Index – Optimize Your Investment

You are the fund manager of your wellness investment portfolio. Invest wisely!

Y ou get to accept the challenge of becoming the fund manager of your *Lifestyle Wellness Index* fund so you can evaluate and balance the ongoing effectiveness of your *Lifestyle Wellness Strategic Plan* through periodic review and evaluation.

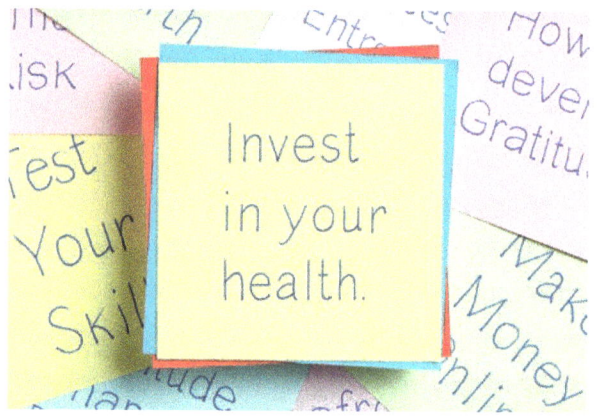

As the fund manager, you periodically evaluate your *LWI*. I recommend weekly reviews for the first two-to-three months so you can reflect, learn, and adapt your tactics, distractions, and tracking processes.

You most likely do this already with new financial investments you make. You first monitor the investment more closely and then may scale back your monitoring later. This also applies to your *Lifestyle Wellness Strategic Plan*.

You get to become your lifestyle wellness index fund manager.

Closer monitoring during the first few months after implementation may help you recognize you want to change your investments or invest more to potentially reduce your chronic disease development risk by moving your goals and targets further toward the green range of the continuum.

Strategic Wellness Activities

The strategic wellness activities in this chapter help you create a measurement plan that includes some basic techniques to measure the implementation and effectiveness of your tactics and distractions and the frequency of measurement—you decide what works for you.

1. Complete the Lifestyle Wellness Index Measurement worksheet.

The measurement worksheet helps you decide the tracking and monitoring tactics that work best for you. Based on the tactics and distractions you've chosen for each lifestyle wellness component, think about the best (and easiest) way(s) and frequency to monitor and maintain your awareness of how you are doing for each component.

2. Complete Section 6.0 My Lifestyle Wellness Index (LWI) Measurement Tactics in your *Lifestyle Wellness Strategic Plan.*

Transcribe your measurement tactics and frequency to monitor and maintain awareness of how you are doing for each component.

Keep your measurements simple and efficient but still able to provide an overview of your progress. In addition, your measurements should give you enough information to decide if you want to adjust your tactics and distractions (investments) to achieve and sustain your long-term wellness transformation.

> NOTE: I suggest using the Perceived Stress Scale, PHQ-2 or PHQ-2 4 for well-being, Connections Quality Evaluation, and Positive Possibilities Mindset Evaluation for your weekly measures.

3. Download and set up your *LWI Statement Tracking Process.*

I've created this spreadsheet for you to monitor and visualize your *Lifestyle Wellness Strategic Plan* performance and return on investment and prepare your monthly and quarterly *LWI Statements.* Follow the instructions in the spreadsheet to get ready to track your mindset progression and progress toward your *Wellness Vision.*

> NOTE: Download the LWI Statement Tracking spreadsheet template in the Week 10 section on the book resource website.

4. Complete the Courage & Confidence Check.

How did you do with creating your measurement plan and preparing yourself to take on your new role of fund manager for your *Lifestyle Wellness Index*? Do your measurement practices reflect your **courage** to maintain a long-term, neutral, and intentional perspective when evaluating your progress toward optimizing your investment in your health and wellness? Lifestyle medicine is about making confident, consistent, forward progress, weathering the ups and downs, and using your *LWI* measurement plan to identify when you must adjust your focus to stay on track with your *Wellness Vision.*

a. You choose the way you want to think and what your progress means to your future wellness. Maintaining a long-term, neutral, and intentional perspective means you don't go negative—all progress is good.

Using a scale of 1-10 (with 10 being Extremely Courageous and 1 being Not Very Courageous At All), how **courageous** are you feeling about implementing your measurement plan and diligently maintaining an investment mindset when evaluating your progress?

My **courage** level:

1   2   3   4   5   6   7   8   9   10

What influenced my rating choice?

_____

_____

If my rating is less than 7, I will take the following actions to increase my **courage** level to implement my measurement plan and stay diligent maintaining my positive mindset when evaluating my progress:

_____

_____

b. You may be used to tracking the minutia to gauge your progress. This is normal with short, get-fit-quick programs and jump-start programs. **Lifestyle wellness is different.** You have the rest of your life as your time horizon. Lifestyle wellness involves a new mindset and way of thinking about your health and wellness, similar to your long-term financial goals.

Keeping your measurement process efficient and aligned with your strengths will improve your **confidence** that you are measuring the right things that gauge your long-term performance.

Using a scale of 1-10 (with 10 being Extremely Confident and 1 being Not Very Confident At All), how **confident** are you about consistently implementing your measurement process to optimize your investment in your health and wellness and achieve the 6-month *Interim Goals* and *Future Targets* you've chosen?

My **confidence** level is:

1   2   3   4   5   6   7   8   9   10

What influenced my rating choice?

_____

_____

If my rating is less than 7, I will take the following actions to continue increasing my **confidence** level to consistently implement my measurement plan to maximize my investment in my health and wellness:

_____

_____

LIFESTYLE WELLNESS INDEX MEASUREMENT WORKSHEET

What you measure you can manage. Evaluating your progress along your wellness journey using daily effectiveness measures provides insight into the impact of your tactics and distractions and your progress toward achieving your *Wellness Vision.*

REMEMBER: **This level of detail is important when you initially implement your** *Lifestyle Wellness Strategic Plan.* **You are experimenting and finding what works and feels authentic to you**. After you find your authenticity and your new beliefs and behaviors become your default go-to, you don't really have to measure, *You Just Know.*

Lifestyle Wellness Components Instructions:

1. Enter your *Interim Goal* for each Lifestyle Wellness component.
2. Develop a daily or weekly measure or rating process to evaluate the percentage level you achieved using your tactics and distractions for each component. Be sure to use the evaluation tools provided on the book resource website.
3. Enter the dates for the week.
4. At the end of each day or a few times each week, take a few moments to reflect and enter the goal percentage you achieved for the day or week.
5. Calculate the WEEK AVE.
6. You will enter your WEEK AVE in the LWI Tracking Spreadsheet.
7. Duplicate this format or create your own format in your planner to document your daily evaluations.

RICE Evaluation Instructions:

1. Enter your *Current Baseline Level* for each RICE component.
2. Enter the dates for the week.
3. At the end of each day or a few times each week, take a few moments to reflect and enter the component rating for the day.
4. Calculate the WEEK AVE.
5. You will enter your WEEK AVE in the LWI Tracking Spreadsheet.
6. Duplicate this format or create your own format in your planner to document your daily evaluations.

EXAMPLE: Your **Nutrition** *Interim Goal* is 60% whole food, plant-based and 70% unsweetened drinks. Identify a way to measure this (i.e., food journal, photos, etc.). Next, enter what you achieved each day that week. Did you achieve 60%, 70%, or 30%. Be honest and candid in your evaluation. The focus is on mindset shift, learning, and growth.

Nutrition Quality Daily Measurement Plan:									
	DATE:								WEEK
ATTRIBUTE	GOAL	SUN	MON	TUE	WED	THUR	FRI	SAT	AVE
Whole-food plant-based (WFPB) meals									
Unsweetened beverages									

Movement Quality Daily Measurement Plan									
	DATE:								WEEK
ATTRIBUTE	GOAL	SUN	MON	TUE	WED	THUR	FRI	SAT	AVE
Structured Movement									
Non-Structured/ Sitting									

Sleep Quality Daily Measurement Plan

ATTRIBUTE	GOAL	SUN	MON	TUE	WED	THUR	FRI	SAT	WEEK AVE
	DATE:								
Wake-Sleep Time									
Sleep Periods									
Sleep-Wake Time									

Stress Management Quality Daily Measurement Plan

ATTRIBUTE	GOAL	SUN	MON	TUE	WED	THUR	FRI	SAT	WEEK AVE
	DATE:								
Healthy Stress Adaption									
Balanced Mental Well-being									

Positivity & Social Connections Quality Daily Measurement Plan:

ATTRIBUTE	DATE: GOAL	SUN	MON	TUE	WED	THUR	FRI	SAT	WEEK AVE
Balanced Meaningful Connections									
Positive Possibilties Mindset									

Risky Substance Avoidance Quality Daily Measurement Plan:

ATTRIBUTE	DATE: GOAL	SUN	MON	TUE	WED	THUR	FRI	SAT	WEEK AVE
Alcohol Avoidance									
Eliminating Tobacco & Other Risky substances									

Supportive Environments Quality Daily Measurement Plan:									
ATTRIBUTE	DATE: **GOAL**	**SUN**	**MON**	**TUE**	**WED**	**THUR**	**FRI**	**SAT**	**WEEK AVE**
Supportive Home Environment									
Supportive Work Environment									

RICE Analysis Measurement Plan:									
At the end of each day, rate each component using the rating scale: Low = 1 to High = 10. Create a *Wellness-Presence* Building Activity for components with a rating less than 7. Goal is to reach and maintain levels greater than 7.									
ATTRIBUTE	DATE: **BASE-LINE**	**SUN**	**MON**	**TUE**	**WED**	**THUR**	**FRI**	**SAT**	**WEEK AVE**
Readiness									
Importance									
Confidence									
Enthusiasm									

NOTES & QUESTIONS TO BE ANSWERED

WEEK 11

A YEAR FROM NOW

There is no end date for working on your health and wellness. You don't get there and then return to your old life.

"The primary reason diseases tend to run in families may be that diets tend to run in families. Ironically, the side effects of eating healthy can be not having to take drugs."

-DR. MICHAEL GREGER

It is almost guaranteed that life will interrupt your health and wellness journey, no matter what you try to do. That's simply part of being human. You now get to prepare yourself to defend against life situations that test your thoughts and beliefs and learn to manage conditions that attempt to disrupt your future focus, motivation, and resilience.

No one can predict the future. That's why your resilience tactics in your *Lifestyle Wellness Strategic Plan* are not future focused but are **feeling-focused**. Different situations can elicit similar feelings and rock our once-solid foundational beliefs. The key is recognizing the feelings, understanding them, and then working through them using your resilience tactics before they lead to lapses and relapses.

In **Week 11**, you get to prepare the **tactics to keep you moving toward your *Wellness Vision*** and the belief in your fantastic wellness future. You didn't put in all the thoughtful effort thus far to risk reverting to old habits that no longer serve you. Use your resilience tactics to build and fortify your natural defenses.

| 18 |

Defending Your Future Focus

Your beliefs are why you do what you do.
Resilience tactics help you identify what will serve
your Wellness Vision now and into the future.

Resilience is about how you **manage and grow through life's challenges**. During times of stress, our subconscious brain takes over. The subconscious brain is the survival brain and seeks pleasure, avoids pain, and conserves energy by recycling old thoughts.

These old thoughts resurface old limitations. **Negativity bias** takes over, and soon you find yourself putting your health and wellness on the back burner.

It doesn't have to be this way. Remember, your thoughts are just sentences in your head. You can stop negative thoughts in their tracks by creating and implementing your *resilience tactics*. **Thinking about and planning for resilience before you need it creates a mindset that supports emotional agility.** You get to equip your conscious brain with the tactics to override your subconscious brain.

Embrace Nonconformity. Defend your wellness with everything you've got!

Stuff will happen. Recognize when your subconscious is trying to derail you. Stay neutral. It's okay that these thoughts resurface; that's part of being human. **What makes the difference is what you do with what you've got.**

136

Strategic Wellness Activities

The strategic wellness activities in this chapter guide you through identifying the thoughts, beliefs, and feelings that may put you at risk for negativity bias that could lead to lapses and relapses along your lifelong strategic wellness journey. You won't identify situations or events but focus on the feelings and emotions that arise when you let your guard down and allow external events, challenges, and circumstances to take over and guide your life. You identify the resilience tactics and support that will keep you on track with your wellness journey when life tries to get in your way.

1. Complete Section 7.0 My Lifestyle Wellness Resilience Tactics section in your *Lifestyle Wellness Strategic Plan.*

Review the **Resilience Checklist** in Section 7.0 and create a *Mindset & Thinking Change Tactic* for each. Use these guidelines to create your tactics.

    a. **Snap your brain out of the current thinking pattern.** Start your tactic with a quick action, sound, or arm/hand motion to stop your emotions in their tracks, such as a finger snap, clap, buzzer noise, or cut motion with your hand.

    b. **Decide how you want to think and what meaning you want.** You decide how to think and what your future holds. If you don't like how you are feeling, change your thoughts to what you want to feel, because you can!

2. Keep your resilience tactics handy for when you need them.

And you will need them. It takes time and practice to implant new mindset and resilience tactics. Until then, write your tactics on a card you keep in your pocket or create a note on your phone.

3. Complete the Courage & Confidence Check.

How do you want to feel living your best life? Did you create effective resilience tactics to stop your brain in its tracks when it starts to go negative? Do your resilience tactics represent the version of you who is **courageous** and **confident** in your investment in a long-term wellness future?

    a. You have the power to create the life you want and walk the wellness talk every day.

Using a scale of 1-10 (with 10 being Extremely Courageous and Confident and 1 being Not Very Courageous and Confident At All), how **courageous** and **confident** are you feeling about implementing your resilience tactics to shift into the new version of you who stays forward and future-focused?

    My **courage** level is:

1   2   3   4   5   6   7   8   9   10

My **confidence** level is:

1   2   3   4   5   6   7   8   9   10

What influenced my rating choices?

_____

_____

If my ratings are less than 7, I will take the following actions to increase my **courage** and **confidence** levels to implement my resilience tactics to shift into the new version of who I am without looking back:

_____

_____

NOTES & QUESTIONS TO BE ANSWERED

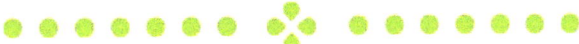

| 19 |

Your Gift to Keep Giving & Getting

Lifestyle wellness is a lifelong journey. Relax, settle in, and enjoy the journey—the ups and downs and all.

Congratulations, you're in the home stretch for completing your *Lifestyle Wellness Strategic Plan.* When you begin implementing your plan, every day is a new day to move forward and progress your Well Leader Mindset™.

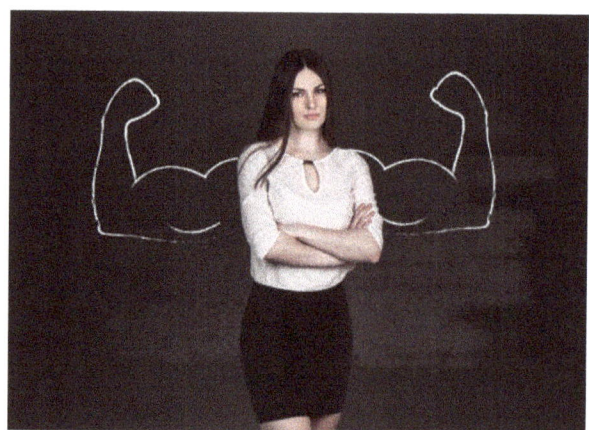

Stay committed and strong; your beliefs guide your actions.

Your beliefs create expectations, and those expectations create your life. Your life is what you expect to find. Your plan helps you practice your beliefs to achieve the expectations of your *Wellness Vision.* Your expectations give you the creative power to stay committed and strong.

Implementing your plan is you simply stepping into the vision of you that you designed in your plan. Implementing your plan is you starting to think, feel, and behave like your *Wellness Vision.* This becomes your new, automatic default, which resides in your subconscious brain, the part that controls 95 percent of your thinking.

Always remember that **your lifestyle wellness is an investment in your future** and something you continue to give yourself and others by creating a ripple effect and paying it forward. It is a work in progress for the rest of your life. So enjoy your incredible wellness journey!

Strategic Wellness Activities

The strategic wellness activities in this chapter put the finishing touches on your plan, so you get to solidify your belief that your *Wellness Vision* is possible now and feel courageous and confident you have a solid path forward.

1. Complete Section 8.0 My Lifestyle Wellness Sustainment Tactics in your *Lifestyle Wellness Strategic Plan.*

Identify and document the next steps and resources to initiate before you implement your plan or engage within the first month. Include due dates to keep yourself on track and add these actions to your calendar. Some examples of next steps may include:

a. Meeting with your family to collaborate on how they can support you, set boundaries and delegate tasks
b. Joining a smoking cessation group in your community
c. Enrolling in a cooking school
d. Ordering a standing desk at work or for your home office
e. Establishing periodic strategic wellness advising sessions with me for ongoing support
f. Joining my Well-Leader Mindset LinkedIn group
g. Enroll in my Well-Leader Mindset - AUTHENTIC Experience, which includes ongoing strategic wellness advising support, certified coaching support, and access to other lifestyle wellness resources.

NOTE: Review the Sustainment Resource & Links located in the Week 11 section on the book resource website.

2. Complete Section 9.0 My Lifestyle Wellness Strategy Planning Insights & Guiding Practices in your *Lifestyle Wellness Strategic Plan.*

Reflect on how your energy, focus, and perceptions have changed as you've moved through this wellness strategic planning process. Record key insights that will guide your thinking, beliefs, and actions going forward.

a. **What is your new forward-focused wellness mindset?**

_____
_____
_____
_____

b. **How will you stay in this mindset and show up for your wellness every day?**

_____

_____
_____
_____
_____

c. **What energy will you bring to your wellness?**

_____
_____
_____
_____

d. **What are your top two guiding principles to keep you focused on your long-term wellness investment?**

_____
_____
_____
_____

3. Complete Section 10.0 My Lifestyle Wellness Strategy Session Insights in your *Lifestyle Wellness Strategic Plan.*

Record your insights and key takeaways from wellness strategy sessions and from collaboration with your Well-Leader peers in my LinkedIn group and group programs. Ongoing engagement will support your forward progress and ensure YOU and your *Lifestyle Wellness Strategic Plan* remain *alive* and *breathing*!

4. Confirm your plan implementation start date.

Demonstrate your formal commitment to **officially implement your *Lifestyle Wellness Strategic Plan*.**

a. Enter your start date in the ***Oath & Commitment to You*** Section. You may have already started implementing some of your tactics and distractions. It's time to get *officially* started when you have your initial external support resources in place.

b. Read your oath out loud, sign it, and date it. This is your official commitment to prioritize and treat you health as an important wealth!

5. Complete the Final Courage & Confidence Check.

How ready are you to step into your authentic wellness and begin living your best life by optimizing your investment in your long-term health and wellness? Are you prepared to accept your lifelong challenge to increase your lifespan and health span?

Did you do the work to feel confident that your completed *Lifestyle Wellness Strategic Plan* represents *you*—the version of you who feels authentic, **courageous**, and **confident** in your ability to invest in your long-term wellness future? This version of you isn't in the distance. That person is right in front of you; step into your authentic wellness!

Using a scale of 1-10 (with 10 being Extremely Courageous and Confident and 1 being Not Very Courageous and Confident At All), how **courageous** and **confident** are you feeling about stepping into the new version of yourself by starting to think, feel, and behave like the new version of who you are?

My **courage** level is:

1   2   3   4   5   6   7   8   9   10

My **confidence** level is:

1   2   3   4   5   6   7   8   9   10

What influenced my rating choices?

_____

_____

If my ratings are less than 7, I will take the following actions to increase my **courage** and **confidence** to implement my plan and step into my authentic wellness by starting to think, feel, and behave like the new version of who I want to be:

_____

_____

NOTES & QUESTIONS TO BE ANSWERED

WEEK 12

MINDSET ALWAYS MATTERS

Show me your wellness, and I will tell you what your beliefs are.

"Setting a goal and slapping actions on it doesn't work; you must change the way you think first."

-LIZ NICKLAS

You are ready to embark officially on your strategic wellness investment journey. You have a solid plan in place and are ready to get started. However, you may still be thinking, what *really* is the point of all the work I completed over the past twelve weeks?

Sure, you are getting your mind organized and creating the plan to live your *Wellness Vision*. But **the true purpose of your work has been to figure out who you are at your authentic best self and become more of that person**. You are unlimited and have no restrictions in terms of the health and wellness you get to create and who you become.

You live in a world of possibility. Nothing is unavailable; however, when you begin blaming others and other things for getting in the way of achieving the health and wellness you desire, you will stay stuck. Even though justification energy feels good and lets you off the hook, it will always be in your way. Unfortunately, this is a human habit we fall into. When you start speaking of your inabilities, limitations, or lack, you create it, choose it, and manifest it.

In **Week 12**, you realize you **have a solid strategy to keep you future-focused.** This strategy allows you to **continually invest in yourself regardless of what is happening in your life.** You now know your health and wellness is not about avoiding struggle. It's about being open to more possibilities. **When your mindset is right, possibility is everywhere.** That's the incredible power of belief.

| 20 |

Well-Leader Mindset – Your New Beginning

Love the process of creating your life and learning while walking through it all. You have limited time on earth, so use every day for learning and leaning into more possibility.

You've reached the end of your lifestyle wellness strategic planning journey and the **beginning of your new life**. Remember, a new beginning always starts with an ending! You must be feeling excited and energized right now – you have a solid strategy and plan to finally achieve and sustain the wellness you desire and start living your best life.

Strategic Wellness Activities

Do you feel the *power* of your new thinking? Don't squander the energy you are feeling right now—get started on your wellness journey today. Don't find yourself a year from now wishing you would have started today!

Commit the **WELL-LEADER MINDSET ™ CREED** to memory. I've included a printable version of the creed on the book resource website for you to download, frame, and hang on your wall. In addition, there is a smaller version for you to print, laminate, and carry with you or snap a photo to use when you need a wellness mindset boost.

1. Reflect on the status of your WELL-LEADER MINDSET™ Strategic Progression

Review each belief in the creed. Then rate each belief from 10-100 percent based on how closely your current thinking aligns. For beliefs rated lower than 70-80 percent alignment, review the associated chapter(s) and strategic wellness activities and schedule a strategy session to achieve clarity and alignment.

WELL-LEADER MINDSET ™ CREED

I Believe:	% Alignment
I have the ability to give myself the gift of health and wellness and that my self-care is a top priority in my life. (Ch 1)	
I am not at the mercy of my genetics; I can and I will control my health and wellness destiny. (Ch 2)	
I have uncovered my true Wellness Why, the Why that controls my thinking, elicits strong positive emotions, and drives my new thoughts and behaviors. (Ch 3)	
I already possess the strengths and values to live my best self; I am confident I know how to use them to strengthen my Wellness Presence and make my wellness journey feel authentic, enthusiastic, and engaging. (Ch 4 & 5)	
I have everything to gain from achieving the long-term health and wellness I desire; I understand the importance of transitioning my beliefs and thinking first before attempting to change my behaviors. (Ch 6 & 7)	
I have a clear, unencumbered Wellness Vision that provides a compelling description of me at my best self; I actively think about my vision every day to change my thinking and change my life; I view failure as an opportunity to learn, expand my possibilities, and achieve even more. (Ch 8 & 9)	
I have aligned my lifestyle wellness strategy with my Wellness Vision. I believe my tactics and distractions are enough to achieve my Future Targets; I can and I will do the work to make my vision a reality. (Ch 10-16)	
My health is as important as my wealth. I treat my strategic lifestyle wellness as a long-term investment in myself and my legacy. I focus on optimizing my return on my wellness investments and monitor and manage my investment wisely. (Ch 17)	
I can manage my external circumstances. I have the power to manage my thoughts and create the experiences I desire. I believe the health and wellness changes I experience create a ripple effect and impact others in positive ways. (Ch 18 & 19)	
It is my duty to live my best life and empower others to better well-being. I believe I am an effective health and wellness role model who advocates for lifestyle wellness at home and in my organization. (Ch 20)	

Which beliefs in the *WLM CREED* did you rate lower than 70-80 percent alignment. What can you do to increase your beliefs alignment for these?

_____

_____

_____

_____

_____

2. Finalize your plan and step into your authentic wellness!

You can, you will, and you get to be the Well-Leader you envision. When you witness yourself stepping forward into your *Wellness Vision*, you not only see yourself differently, but you also change your life.

When you control your thinking and actions, you give yourself the personal power to achieve your vision, despite what is going on in the external world. Your successful transformation to a WELL-LEADER MINDSET™ occurs first at the thought and feeling level of your brain, and then authentic actions follow.

3. Recite the *WELL-LEADER MINDSET ™ CREED* daily and whenever you feel your courage and confidence wane.

The creed continues to solidify your new beliefs and thinking in your subconscious and crowd out old, limiting thoughts. Keeping the creed in view reminds you that your new beliefs and thinking are driving your behaviors—not the media, other people, or external events.

You can't control these; you can only control how you think about them. This keeps your emotions in check and allows you to take action that supports your health and wellness every day. Your beliefs and thinking help you "Be It" first in your mind, then "Do It," and then "Have It," so you experience the outcomes you desire.

4. Download and print the *WELL-LEADER MINDSET ™ CREED* for framing and to use as a pocket card.

NOTE: Download the print versions in the Week 12 section on the book resource website.

NOTES & QUESTIONS TO BE ANSWERED

EPILOGUE Join Me In My Future Pull

Our decisions decide our destiny. Where will your decisions take you?

My incredible thought leader coach Sara Connell said that miraculous future pulls accelerate *Yeses.* They do so by giving you the feelings, thoughts, and most importantly, sensations **as if it is already happening or done**.

Every day **future-pull yourself toward the health and wellness you desire**. Send yourself messages from a virtual coach or someone who would motivate you and pull you forward.

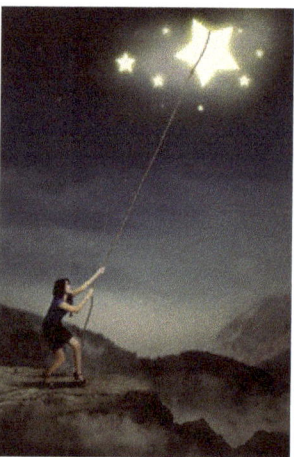

Be your future Now!

Strategic Wellness Activities

One more future pull for the road ahead.

1. Choose an area or goal that feels challenging for you.
2. State your goal as if it is already done.
3. Talk with yourself, a friend, or a support group about the goal as if it has already manifested.
4. Notice the sensations and feelings in your body.
5. Proceed with your day as if your goal has already happened.

Use this format and fill in the blanks.

"**What an amazing day. I've achieved** <your goal>. **It feels** <describe your feelings in a way you feel it in your body>. **I am most excited about** <describe what excites you the most about achieving this goal>. **Now that I've achieved** <restate your goal>, **I get to** <describe how you will be and act going forward and what is next for you>. The future is mine!"

Look for evidence to validate you have achieved your goal. For example, if you see someone else's success story, use it as a sign that it will happen to you. Reality will catch up when you believe into your future and take inspired action.

YOUR JOURNEY FORWARD

Go forth; your endless wellness possibilities await!

"Be the well-leader you've always wanted to meet, and share your wellness legacy now - pay it forward!"

-DR. LORI LINDBERGH

So that's it. By creating your *Lifestyle Wellness Strategic Plan*, you are ready to begin your journey. You've *taken the time to take the time* to think strategically about your long-term investment in your health and wellness.

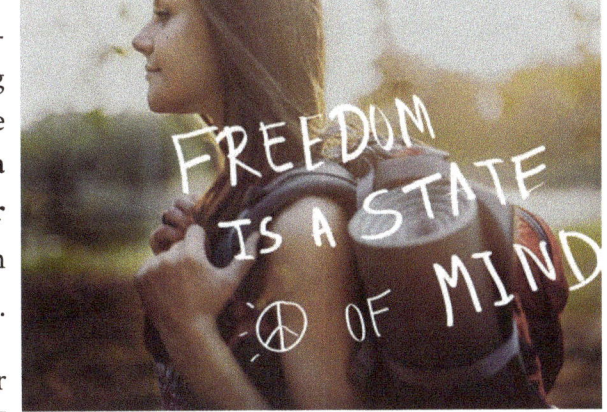

I guarantee that if you were thoughtful and candid in your evaluations, reflections, and planning activities, and you have practiced shifting your mindset using the courage and confidence checks, **you can, and you will experience a level of health and wellness you've never achieved before** as you continue to invest in your wellness and implement your lifelong plan.

You put in the thoughtful work to create your path to step into your **authentic wellness**. I am so excited for you to get started on your journey. I've been where you are now. I know the incredible wellness that you get to create for yourself.

You get to feel the freedom. *Wellness Freedom* is a state of mind. No more beating yourself up, and no more *shoulding* and *shouldn'ting* all over yourself! You have **eliminated your wellness cognitive dissonance** and quieted your mind. You are no longer stuck in a cycle of wellness failure.

You get to live your lifestyle of wellness and show up as your best self every day. Continue your focus on mindset shift and growth. There will be ups and downs; accept progress and growth, not perfection.

By implementing your plan, you get to shift effortlessly into achieving your *Wellness Vision*! You are resilient, and you get to invest in the support you desire. Your work and home environments are set up to support your success.

Endless possibilities lie ahead for you. You are well on your way to membership in *The 3% Club!* Stay connected with me and other Well-Leaders to keep your momentum going and grow the movement.

- **Connect with me and other Well-Leaders** on LinkedIn and join my LinkedIn group: Well-Leader Mindset – The 3% Club
- **The book resource website is a wealth of health information.** Check back for updated resources and tips often.
- **Take your wellness journey to the next level.** Join my **WELL-LEADER MINDSET™ – Authentic** program. Get expert support and collaboration to implement your *Lifestyle Wellness Strategic Plan* and continue your journey down your authentic path to wellness. Use the link in the Week 12 section on the book resource portal and find out more on my website: www.loriuslifestyle.com.
- **Feel free to schedule a 1-on-1 Wellness Strategy Session** with me when you need a little extra support. Use the link in the Week 12 section on the book resource website to schedule a session.
- **Join the biweekly group strategy sessions.** The main page of the book resource website contains the link to join the group sessions.

It has been an honor to support you along this part of your strategic wellness investment journey. I love to support leaders with strategizing and planning for extraordinary health and wellness.

The next steps to optimizing your health and wellness ROI by stepping into your authentic wellness are yours to take. Along the way, stay connected and always reach out when you need support. I will be here when you need me.

Here's to your authentic wellness future for life.

Lori

Dr. Lori Lindbergh considers herself a disruptor, innovator, and nonconformist throughout her diverse career as a registered nurse, healthcare leader, performance consultant, industrial/organizational psychologist, and now as a **Wellness Investment Strategist**.

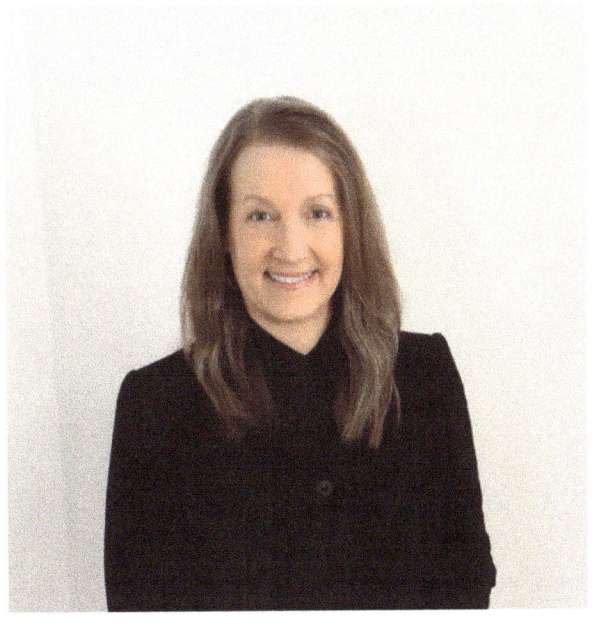

Lori was a self-proclaimed unwell leader for over thirty years until she experienced her wake-up call and cracked the wellness code. Her book, inspired by her journey and that of her late father, a decorated WWII veteran, transforms readers into savvy *Wellness Investors* who learn to treat their health as important as their wealth using the proprietary process in her book and this investment guide. Until now, there has been no evidence-based framework to do so.

Lori hopes that by helping leaders live well and lead well, they will walk-the-wellness-talk and empower their people at work and home to value wellness and embark on their wellness journeys. Leaders have a duty to pay it forward and make a difference in the well-being of others.

Dr. Lori Lindbergh, Wellness Investment Strategist

Lori is a Board Certified Lifestyle Medicine Professional through the American College of Lifestyle Medicine, National Board Certified Health & Wellness Coach (NBC-HWC), Mayo Clinic Certified Wellness Coach, and Certified in Whole Food, Plant-Based Nutrition through eCornell University. **She specializes in executive and leadership wellness investing and organizational wellness culture transformation.**

Her innovative, client-focused, strategic **wellness investment framework** integrates mindset and behavior change strategies, strategic leadership practices, evidence-based lifestyle medicine guidelines, and wellness coaching practices within an investment context to help executives and leaders find their *authentic wellness for life* and translate that into improved support for well-being in their organizations.

Learn more about Lori's WELL-LEADER MINDSET™ **Strategic Progression Framework** and **Wellness Investing Programs** at www.loriuslifestyle.com. Contact her by email at lori@loriuslifestyle.com and connect via LinkedIn.

ACKNOWLEDGEMENTS

My life would not be where it is without the tireless, noble work of the American College of Lifestyle Medicine (ACLM). They are on a mission to change the delivery of healthcare and improve the healthcare status of the world.

Many chronic diseases of lifestyle are preventable and reversible by changing our health behaviors and actions. ACLM is that consistent voice that provides the evidence and resources for providers to guide the changes that will add years to your life and life to your years. Visit ACLM at lifestylemedicine.org to view resources and find a board-certified provider to support your wellness journey.

www.ingramcontent.com/pod-product-compliance
Lightning Source LLC
Chambersburg PA
CBHW041535120626
46551CB00019B/2711